Cancer

How You, Your Marriage, Family and Business Can Survive and Thrive Through Cancer Diagnosis, Treatment and Recovery

1.23

By   Koenigs

13-Time #   selling Author

Free Canc   Videos

This book include   os and interviews with
survivors that ca   p you or a loved one
navigate through   omplex challenges of
living with and s   ing cancer with your
marriage, family and business intact.

Go here: www.Cancerpreneur.com

Free and Frequent Updates!

I'm frequently updating this book with more interviews, resources and information based on the feedback you share and I'm always adding new information from survivors, doctors and health professionals I meet and talk to.

If you are reading this book on a Kindle or Kindle App, make sure it's the latest version.

To get the latest and greatest, just open your app, click or press the "More" icon in the lower right-hand corner and then press "Sync" and you'll always be up to date. See the image below.

I appreciate comments and feedback so head over to www.YEN.tv/CancerpreneurReview right now!

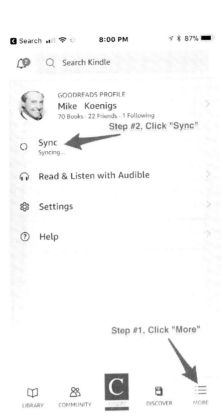

Step #2, Click "Sync"

Step #1, Click "More"

To my incredible wife, my Queen, Vivian—
You're my conscience.

And my son, Zak—
You amplify my gratitude to be alive.

I love both of you so much.
You are my universe.

My family and friends, I'll mention all of you in the next
edition of this book and give you the credit you deserve.

Dr. Worsey, Dr. Bannerjee, and Dr. Christopher Willett
Thank you for saving my life.

Dr. Nalini Chilkov and JJ Virgin—
Thank you for bringing me back to life.

To my amazing customers—
Thank you for believing in me while I was down for the
count and couldn't get up on my own.

100% of the money earned from this book is donated to
the Just Like My Child Foundation, a 501c3 nonprofit.
www.JustLikeMyChild.org

Disclaimer

I want to help you survive and thrive. Having said that, I'm not a doctor. I don't play one on the Internet or on TV, so consult your medical doctor for health advice.

Please seek medical supervision before attempting to do anything recommended in this book. If there's a tiebreaker to be made, don't listen to me. Trust your instincts.

Don't do anything stupid with yours or someone else's life.

Table of Contents

Who Am I and Why Should You Listen to Me?

"Get that thing cut out of you and get your life in order—or you're a dead man in less than six months."

I was an idiot ... for six months.

I started bleeding from my butt and didn't do anything about it ... until it was too late. I started noticing spots of blood in the toilet and later, spots of blood on every chair when I sat down. I started wearing black underwear and pants, so I wouldn't think about it. My dad suffered from hemorrhoids, so did I, and occasionally they bled. That's what I thought I had—bleeding hemorrhoids—which I ignored. Looking back, I knew something was wrong, but like many busy entrepreneurs say: "I just don't have time to slow down. My business will fall apart. That'll never happen to me."

Yeah right. After ignoring the problem and seeing it worsen over months, I confessed to my wife, Vivian, that I was bleeding when I pooped.

Her response was as subtle as a landmine: "People who bleed out of their ass have cancer, Mike. Go to the doctor." (My wife is a nice Jewish girl from New York who grew up in Manhattan. No, not that Manhattan. Spanish Harlem. "Subtle" isn't in the vocabulary when it comes to discussing health in our family. ;))

I made an appointment to have a colonoscopy. I missed the first one and the next available appointment was two months later. Not good.

Two months later after the rescheduled exam, the doctor delivered some ugly words: "You have a 5.5-centimeter tumor, located right above the top of your rectum and at the end your lower sigmoid colon. Get that thing cut out of you, get your life in order, or you're a dead man in less than six months."

On my end—fear. Utter fear. On top of that, I had to tell my family.

I got it together and flew to Minnesota to tell my parents and three siblings in person, to let them know that I was going to undergo surgery and I wasn't sure what was going to happen next.

◆ ◆ ◆

A week later, surgery. Right before I was put under, I instructed the doctor, "If you have to give me a colostomy bag, don't bother waking me up. I'd rather be dead."

My biggest fears at that time, especially given the fact that I had colon cancer, were that I'd lose the ability to have sex or I'd lose my sex drive; I'd be stuck with a stinky colostomy bag the rest of my life; and/or I'd be crippled in some other ludicrous way.

When I woke after the surgery, the first thing I did was reach down. Yes! No colostomy bag! And the surgery seemed to have gone well.

But …

The following day, the surgeon, armed with a biopsy report, informed me that several of my lymph nodes were cancerous. That put me at stage 3a. What this meant: I was a "perfect" candidate for chemotherapy treatments and very possibly radiation too. Fortunately the cancer hadn't spread to my organs, bones, or broken through the colon wall (or I'd be stage 4, which is often fatal or has an extremely high rate of recurrence).

On my horizon then were lengthy, involved, and uncomfortable (to put it mildly) treatments. But, if this extended my life, I was in. My 10-year-old son needed his daddy. And my nice Jewish wife would be really pissed if I checked out too soon. :)

Why me? Why cancer? What contributed to that fateful day when the doctor dropped the bomb on me, the bomb I'd been denying for 6+ months? Ultimately it was a combination of an intense lifestyle, an enormous amount of stress, and a failure to heed multiple warnings until it was too late.

My background is pretty typical for a hard-driving entrepreneur. I was raised in a lower middle-class home in Eagle Lake, Minnesota, where it was cold, and I mean really cold, like 35 degrees below zero kind of cold. My dad worked really hard as a barber. Also he worked as Eagle Lake's City Clerk, Building Inspector, and the guy who did lots of other little jobs to make ends meet. My mom was at home with us four kids and worked part-time at the Catholic school we went to. Because my dad worked so much, we were usually late and last for everything.

I spent most of my youth angry and frustrated, feeling not good enough and being tortured and terrorized by bullies on a school bus filled with children of the '60s and '70s. I HATED school, starting on day one. I sure as hell never hid that fact from anyone. I became an altar boy as a means of skipping school. I barely passed high school. I never went to college.

What I remember most from my childhood was being cold a lot of the time. Being cold pissed me off, so that contributed to me being mad and frustrated. I always knew I wanted to work with computers and taught myself how to program when I was 14. Unfortunately, owning a computer was out of the question. The most common phrase heard in our home was: "We can't afford it." So if you asked me what I wanted to be when I grew up, the answer was "Rich, first and warm."

I kept a backpack in my closet packed with my belongings and fantasized about running away from home to Palo Alto, California, to work for Apple Computer for Steve Jobs and Steve Wozniak. I figured that would never happen, so to achieve my "rich, first and warm" dream, I drove myself really hard. I started working full-time on my 16th birthday. I started writing software professionally at age 19. In my early 20s, I started and sold a business, made a movie, and taught myself online marketing. I married my high-school sweetheart, got divorced, and lived the up-and-down life of an entrepreneur. I didn't stop for much of a break—until that fateful day.

Working so hard for so long did get me the wealth, the warmth (I moved to San Diego), and (some of) the security I yearned for in my youth. Becoming a bit of a celebrity in my business sector gave me a degree of VIP status and made me "first" most of the time. But there's always a flipside.

Less-than-ideal habits often accompany super hard work and big ambitions. Part of growing up in a small, lower middle-class community in Minnesota meant that I was legally able to drink at 18. It was part of our culture, so for the majority of my adult life, I'd drink a couple times per week. On top of that, I had poor eating behaviors, mostly because I just didn't know any better and I never took the time to learn. And as far learning how to manage that anger I had since childhood, it was never a priority. I was always occupied with my entrepreneurial initiatives...and subconscious fears that were eating me alive.

As time went on, my big aspirations and growing success reaped a full life. Along with the fame, luxuries and splendor was a ton of stress, lots of travel, moving really fast, and living in the tomorrow instead of the now. My focus was on the future and on more - because my biggest fear was running out and not having enough.

The ugly words the doctor delivered that fateful day are what brought my fast-lane living to an abrupt halt. It's nothing short of a miracle how that ugly opening to a horrific year ended up giving me a new beginning—a new beginning that I had no idea how much I was in desperate need of.

Cancer changed my life. Correction. Cancer saved my life.

A Message from Mike's Wife, Vivian

No one invites cancer into their life.

Yet, a cancer diagnosis is an offer to embark on a spiritual journey, an offer you can't refuse. Your attendance is required. There's no postponing or rescheduling for another time that's more convenient.

And it's not just required attendance for you (the person who is diagnosed)—your entire family must attend as well. Immediately.

My husband's cancer diagnosis came at a most inconvenient time. His business was on the rocks. He was going through a massive mid-life crisis that some days made me just want to kill him myself, and on other days, made me terrified for the future of our family. Our 10-year-old needed his daddy's attention more than ever. My non-profit organization, Just Like My Child, was like another child, calling for constant, never-ending attention.

The invitation came in the form of rectal bleeding that persistently beckoned us to the spiritual path. It couldn't be cajoled to pipe itself down. It wouldn't be postponed to another day. The more we ignored it, the more urgent the invitation became.

Looking back, this unwelcome invitation came at the perfect time.

In the months leading up to Mike's diagnosis he was angry and stressed—at times unbearable. I couldn't do anything right. Like a typical co-dependent, I stayed because I felt somehow responsible for his behavior. As in: "If only I can work out my own issues and be more perfect, then he won't be such a jerk." I found the love I needed in my son and in my work.

The diagnosis came at the moment when he and I together had to stop and face the demons that were making us miserable, head-on. Through our own insecurities, unresolved childhood wounds, and resulting imperfections, we had to summon the beast inside of ourselves.

We had to find the compassion, love, courage, resourcefulness, and integrity of character to bring to the fight for survival. The journey through cancer requires nothing less, and as we had unconsciously succumbed to the stressors of life, we were woefully unprepared.

Cancer's invitation, this visit from the angel of death itself, saved our marriage, saved our family, saved our businesses, and saved our very souls. It redefined the container of marriage that we inhabit every day.

When Mike was diagnosed with colorectal cancer, he was young, vibrant, healthy. He was full of energy and resourcefulness, and had led a pretty healthy life.

I'll never forget that moment when his surgeon came into the hospital room after she had cut out a large tumor from his gut and the cells had gone through pathology. We had been led to believe that maybe he could just have the tumor removed, recover from surgery, and get up and walk away from the hospital bed without looking back.

She had tears in her eyes as she said, "I went back to the lab twice and looked myself. I didn't believe that it was true, I was so hoping that it wasn't going to turn out this way, but you have stage 3a cancer. Your lymph is involved. You are invited to the full-meal deal: chemotherapy and possible radiation. It's your best chance for survival."

The reality that he might not survive had walked into the room with her. The big bony finger of this beckoning invitation popped through our delicate structure of certainty and demanded that we step onto cancer's spiritual path, without any possibility of turning back.

Welcome to Cancerpreneur

This book represents five incredibly challenging and rewarding years on a journey through cancer and recovery. It's an experience that I hope I will never have to relive, but I'm incredibly grateful for having done so.

My goal for this book is simple: to help you or someone you care about survive and thrive after being diagnosed with cancer and getting treated for it. My aim is to simplify the confusing journey, so you'll experience a lot less pain, hardship, confusion, and overwhelm than *what I—and my family—endured.*

My book will help you save time and simplify the experience so that your encounter with cancer can be as clear and painless as possible, with the fewest number of complications and side effects as possible, and with all of your most significant relationships—and your business— completely intact.

In fact, I feel completely comfortable promising that you will emerge from this experience a better person than when you begin. Hindsight is powerful medicine, and anyone who's made it to the other side always agrees that cancer is a great teacher and you're wiser than when you began.

If you have short attention or ADD (like me) or you learn better and faster with videos, then go to www.Cancerpreneur.com where you can watch several transformational survivor and doctor interviews and access powerful healing tools and resources.

I created this book for you—if you've been diagnosed with cancer; if you, a loved one, a spouse, a child, a friend, or a colleague has been diagnosed with cancer; or if you are a business owner and want to know how to prepare yourself, so you either don't get cancer or can deal with it in case it happens.

After going through this process myself and serving as an advisor to hundreds of friends, family members, and business associates that call me for my perspective, advice, and feedback on their encounters with cancer, I feel absolutely confident in sharing all I've learned. It's the stuff that matters.

Here's what you can expect from this book and the additional bonus video content, so you get the most out of it in the shortest period of time.

First, it's interactive. There are lots of opportunities for you to go deeper into the content and gain access to the free videos, resources, and other tools that I've provided.

Second, this book is intended to help you or your loved one survive—with no BS. I have no hidden agenda. My single incentive is to share my experience, my "version of the truth" to make sure you or someone you care about survives.

Third, it's for people who want to live and are interested in survival—no matter what it takes. I take on controversial points of view in this book, and at times it may push your belief systems. I'm not here to make you comfortable or to be your best friend, I'm interested in results. In other words, I'm not on anyone's side except survival's. So, if you already have a preconceived notion of what you think is right or wrong in terms of cancer treatments and recovery, then you might as well just be right and close this book right now.

However, if you want no BS and simple truth from a survivor who has interviewed and talked to hundreds of doctors and worked as a medical industry marketer talking to good and bad doctors alike, I can give you a fresh perspective.

My book comes from the point of view of a survivor who walked into cancer with a damaged marriage that is now stronger than it's ever been in 16 years and who now has a remarkable and connected relationship with his 15-year-old son.

Plus, I managed to not only have my business survive and thrive while facing cancer, but I was able to package and sell it to a publicly traded company. Every one of my personal and business relationships are stronger now than ever before.

I will also add that my relationship with my entire family of two living parents and three siblings has greatly improved.

Fourth, this book isn't intended to be a New York Times #1 bestseller. It's designed to start a conversation with you, to give you and me a chance to get to know each other better and develop a bond, and ultimately, to give you the tools, knowledge, and resources to survive or help someone you care about survive.

Fifth, this book is short, but packed with easy-to-implement recommendations and lots of ideas. My intention is to give you hope, to inspire you, motivate you, and give you needed clarity, focus and knowledge, so you can make clear decisions without feeling as though you have to second guess yourself throughout a complex process that often results in permanent damage or death.

I'll be the first to admit that I am opinionated. I have strong ideas, but all of them are backed up with a significant amount of research, results, and my own survival.

If you like what's in this book, I'd absolutely, positively love to hear from you, get to know you better, and have you share your success story, your transformation, your picture or a video, and comment on my Facebook wall at www.Facebook.com/Koenigs.

The best way to start a relationship with me will be to visit the link in this book at www.Cancerpreneur.com and get the free videos. Feel free to share this book with anyone you know who is in need of a transformation in their survival.

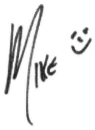

Sincerely,
Mike Koenigs
La Jolla, California, USA

P.S. I wrote and edited this book myself and with the help of a couple special people in less than a week. There are absolutely, positively some spelling, grammatical, and lay-out errors. If you find one, will you do me a favor, and sending me an email to MikeKoenigs@gmail.com? Note the page number, sentence, and mistake, and I'll fix it right away. Thank you for your help in advance. I'm all about results, implementation, and speed, and I've chosen to give you a resource that will help save a life, rather than attempt to land perfection.

P.P.S. If you love this book or you've found it helps you or someone you care about, will you please post a review on Amazon at www.YEN.tv/CancerpreneurReview? Nothing will make me happier than to hear your personal transformation survival story and your feedback.

P.P.P.S. If you don't like this book, will you please just send me an email and tell me why? I will gladly give you your money back. Please be kind. I have a son. He reads what people say about me online and so do his friends! There's no sense in posting a nasty, negative comment and dragging an innocent kid into something unnecessary.

My Responsibility to You

As a cancer survivor I feel like I have a responsibility to share what I learned with anyone who's diagnosed with cancer. Over the past five years since I've recovered, I have been getting calls from friends, friends of friends, family, friends of family, and business associates seeking my advice. Most of the time the advice I give is exactly the same. That's why I wrote this book.

What I'm including in this book is what to expect from cancer and how I believe you should take it on: how to survive, how to deal with the onslaught of "help" that you're going to get from other people, and how to manage the information that gets thrown at you. Trust me, people from all over the place are going to call you to "help," thinking that they're the only one who's providing it to you. There is a strategy in how to determine what is real and what is not real, which I'll share. I'm going to guide you through the emotional and the physical trauma that you are likely to experience as well.

Now a few quick words if you don't have cancer. Statistically speaking, one in two men are diagnosed with cancer sometime during their lives, and one in three women. So if it doesn't directly happen to *you*, it certainly will happen to *someone you know*. For this reason you should get prepared to have a conversation, to deal with the trauma, and to address all the questions that pop up.

If you are the person who just found out you have cancer, I'm going to give you a zero BS, no sugar-coated, just-the-facts-as-I-see-them strategy to surviving and thriving. If you or someone you know has cancer, the biggest thing that I found is you (or they) will want a combination of hope and clarity.

Recently I got a call from a friend who's been diagnosed with stage 4 colorectal cancer (I had stage 3a, which means it got to my lymph, but not into my bones and organs). His doctor told him he had a 0% chance of survival, which, if you think about it, seems cruel and inhumane. I guess it's necessary for a doctor to tell their version of the truth, but none of us wants to feel as though we are nothing more than a statistic without hope.

I know people who are living and walking miracles. They've survived for years with stage 4 cancer and are not cancer-free. I think it's important that you have hope that maybe you might be one of the miracles also. That way you don't just curl up in a ball and give up.

Having no hope is not fair to you, your family and the people who love you. In this book, in addition to telling you how cancer can play out, I'll give you hope, no matter how dire the prognosis.

The next thing that's important is survival. Information, resources, and conversing with an informed group to share these things are key to surviving. In this book you'll find links and information on how to contact me and follow me on Facebook and social media, so we can create a flow of information and share stories to support one another's survival. I want to hear your transformational and survival story.

I've had the good opportunity to present in front of thousands of survivors. I've spoken to lots of doctors. Because of the nature of my business, I have an enormous number of clients and customers who are in the healing practices industry: doctors, nutritionists, fitness experts, and lots of New York Times bestselling authors who are considered some of the biggest thought leaders in the health and healing professions.

The reason I'm telling you this is when I provide support, information, recommendations, and resources in this book, I'm doing so from a place of substantive evidence. Of course, we are all subject to confirmation bias, meaning we typically seek out information that supports the beliefs that we already have. Even still, for you to heal, for you to grow as a result of cancer and be able to look back at it in the future and call it the greatest gift you've ever received in your life, it is crucial that you are willing to test your notion of reality. It is essential you hear things that make you feel flat out uncomfortable and stretch yourself in new directions. That's how you'll grow. That's how you'll not only survive but also thrive.

Without further ado, let's dive right in.

The Essential Elements for Survival

To be prepared for war is one of the most effective means of preserving peace.

—George Washington

When people seek my recommendations for surviving cancer, there's certain things I always say. That's what I'm giving here in this chapter: the essential elements for survival.

Stay the Course

Listen to and follow the advice of your doctors.

Why am I telling you this? Let me give you the backstory. I regularly receive calls from friends who have started cancer treatments. They may have gotten diagnosed. Maybe they had surgery, or they didn't yet have surgery. And they got through one or two of their treatments. Then they decide that they are going to call it quits. Why? The Internet.

They start finding all kinds of horror stories on the Internet of people talking about how their doctors are full of it and the companies that make cancer-related drugs have a massive conspiracy running to get money and kill people.

That simply isn't the case.

Google doesn't cure cancer. The Internet is filled with advice from people who know nothing about medicine, who post anything they want, and who won't go to jail if they give you bad information or if you die.

So, the first and most important lesson: you need to find doctors and health professionals *that you feel are competent.* And, when you learn how to ask them really good questions, which I'm going to address later in this book, you can survive. You can beat all the odds.

In my opinion, cancer survival is partially a game of statistics. It's important to know what medical facts are statistically relevant and accurate for someone like you with the condition you have.

Once you understand this, it isn't necessarily important that you subscribe to all the data and evidence. What is important is that you have some solid information to help you make some good decisions. For example, if you gather some evidence-based information that the treatment that's been prescribed to you has a 0% chance of working, then it doesn't make a lot of sense to go through with it. Similarly, if you find out that, statistically speaking, the treatment has a 100% chance of working, and the risk of not using it could kill you, you'd be a fool not to take advantage of that.

It is important that you take these findings into account, so you can navigate the huge volumes of information that are going to be thrown at you. And you should expect a lot of information to come your way.

The other thing to take into account is even before you start any treatment, you will feel fatigued. You will feel tired. You will experience information overload and overwhelm. Unless you have someone very close to you navigating with you every step of the way, it's important that you have a system and a process to help you survive.

Your Golden Goose

Your golden goose, or rather, geese, are nurses.

As soon as I received my cancer diagnosis and I went through surgery, I started watching and paying attention to nurses. I was amazed at how they took on my illness and were able to be cheerful and fulfilled even though they were surrounded by people that might not be alive next month.

After dealing with many doctors (I'll address them shortly), I learned that they don't always tell you exactly what they think and exactly what they should tell you simply because they are working for a corporation, a hospital. The nurses, on the other hand, have some great insights and can be more candid once you get into rapport with them.

I got into the habit of asking almost every nurse that I worked with a few simple questions. The primary question: how accurate are you at being able to predict, for a person with cancer, who survives and who dies?

Invariably the experienced ones who I knew had wisdom beyond their years would smile and confide that they could almost always tell. They explained that the people who survive are the ones who take on their cancer. Who go to battle with it. Who take all the tools and resources in their reach, and use all of them all at once. More than one nurse called it "going thermonuclear."

The people who die are the people who blame other people. They complain. They take on a bad attitude or a victim mentality. They hesitate, or they are indecisive. The nurses consistently said your decisiveness will determine whether you live or die.

My greatest advice to you is find and speak to the nurses that you genuinely feel are fully involved in their work. They're the ones with great attitudes. They have experience, I'm talking 15–20+ years of experience. (Obviously, you don't want to take advice from someone who's brand-new, has a bad attitude, or clearly doesn't want to be there because they're not invested in your survival or in their careers.)

Armchair Quarterbacks—Benched

Next up, what I have found consistently helps is being part of a support group, whether that is a teaming up with a supportive family member or with survivors.

I turn off the noise and do not take advice from people who don't have skin in the game. In other words, if they don't have something to lose. For example, the doctor that consistently provides bad advice or who routinely has patients die probably isn't going to be in the profession very long.

Don't take advice from people who haven't been through what you've been through. You don't want an armchair quarterback coaching your game.

You want to talk to real survivors who had what you have and can tell you what the good, the bad, and the ugly really is.

Full Disclosure Always

Do what the doctors tell you, and don't hide what you're doing from them either.

For example, if your oncologist tells you to do something, do it. And if they tell you, for example, to not take supplements while you are doing chemotherapy, don't take supplements. Supplements will counteract the effect of chemotherapy and may end up causing an incredible amount of damage to you if take them while getting chemotherapy treatment.

Ear Plugs Please

Here's a list of things you don't want to listen to.

Don't listen to the Internet.

Unless you are an expert researcher, you want to be very careful about what you believe and what you encounter, especially if you can't verify the sources.

Don't listen to MLM or network marketing organizations.

I was amazed and surprised at the number of people who came out of the woodwork when they found out that I was diagnosed with cancer touting all sorts of potions, lotions, creams, pills, and solutions that would supposedly heal my cancer. They were nobodies from nowhere that wanted to profit from my sickness.

While I say to avoid these "magic pill pushers," you'll find out later, I'm not at all opposed to or against using high-quality supplements and resources, as long as you've discussed them with your doctors. However, you want to be careful about listening to people who won't go to prison for giving you bad advice.

Don't listen to the fuzzy bunnies.

There will be all sorts of woo-woo folks who believe in unicorns, fairy tales, fuzzy bunnies, feathers, and crystals, and they will want to heal you.

Shortly after I was diagnosed, I got 11 second opinions. Out of those 11, one was from a very well known nutrition "doctor" (he had an MD on his wall) who was a proponent of alkaline diets, coffee enemas, juice enemas, and using a variety of light therapy and other integrative therapies that were unproven and unregulated. That person told me that he thought I shouldn't do any treatments at all: no surgery, no chemotherapy, and no radiation.

Exactly three months after he gave me that horrible advice that I ignored, that person was arrested and prosecuted for practicing medicine without a license in the state of California. Ultimately he went to prison.

If I had listened to him, I believe I would be dead. Of the other 10 people I got advice from, some were proponents and practitioners of alternative and integrative medical treatments, and some of them were traditional allopathic doctors. All advised me to get treatment.

My point is there are crazy people who are unlicensed and often have profit as their motive. Or they're just nuts. They can kill you if you listen to them.

Zero to a Thousand ASAP

You want to "go thermonuclear" right away.

The moment you find out what you have, you want to use every tool and resource at your disposal to get rid of it. In my experience, the people who hesitate or second guess are the ones who are dead.

Play the stats game right from the start. The stats don't have to be your final decision, but they are important for making good decisions.

My advice is to use all the allopathic resources at your fingertips right away. Meet with an alternative or integrative doctor as quickly as possible to do supplemental therapies that prevent damage and degradation to your body while you're getting treated. Once your primary treatments are done, use alternative and integrative systems to heal and return to normalcy.

What is crucial is not to quit or just do it halfway. Those people end up crippled or dead.

No Cape and Tights

Don't be a hero and resist taking painkillers.

Looking back, I did not take painkilling drugs as quickly as I should have or could have to reduce the pain. As a result, an enormous amount of trauma started happening to my brain and body because, like the frog in the pan that gets heated up and the frog eventually boils to death, I got used to the pain.

I'm not telling you to just take a ton of drugs, nor am I recommending you do so. All I'm saying is I've met a lot of people who "muscle through the pain" for months, and I can just tell they're miserable and don't have to be that way. If you're an addict and have addictive behaviors, I'm not speaking to you :) Everything in moderation.

Based on my personal experience and from talking to other survivors, doctors, and other professionals in the healing arena, the brain and body heal at different rates. If your body is in constant pain, it causes emotional trauma and vice-versa. Your body and brain need an opportunity to rest—and because they are "separate," they need to be treated as such.

With that in mind, when you take painkillers, your brain doesn't experience the body's pain, so it can rest. Similarly when you don't experience the waves of pain and you aren't focused on it, your body isn't tense and in a constant state of tension, so it can rest too. My advice is take the painkilling drugs, so your brain and your body can heal, and it will reduce your trauma as well.

Plan on your recovery process taking you a year. Recovery takes time, and the trauma is deeper than you can imagine.

Survival: A 5-Ingredient Recipe

When I asked doctors, this simple question—how can you tell if someone is going to survive or die?—they answered by pointing out what they saw in me. You'll notice it's similar to how the nurses answered the same question.

- *Ingredient 1*: I always saw you with a smile on your face.
- *Ingredient 2*: You never made your process about anything except getting well. You were never a victim.
- *Ingredient 3*: You took interest in what was going on. You were absolutely committed to your survival.
- *Ingredient 4*: You took full responsibility for everything that was happening, and you changed your behavior and mindset to make sure everything worked out. In other words, you were coachable and willing to examine anything that threatened an old belief system you had.
- *Ingredient 5*: You did everything in your power without hesitation to eliminate and kill the disease.

I believe this is the recipe for survival. When people ask me, "How did you survive cancer and what advice can you give me or someone I care about who was recently diagnosed?" it's these five things that I make sure to tell them.

Up next: we explore the relationship between your emotional self and cancer. Emotions likely played a part in getting cancer, and they certainly play a part in beating it.

Why Did You Get Cancer and Does It Matter?

Disease is, in essence, the result of conflict between soul and mind, and will never be eradicated except by spiritual and mental effort.
—Edward Bach

What I share in this chapter might be controversial, but it matters. It's a question that I ask every person who I talk to who has undergone cancer: "Why did you get cancer and does it matter anyway?" I then go on to connect the answers to this question to the mindset I recommend adapting to aid in the healing process.

The Emotional Factor

There's a book by the great late Louise Hay called *You Can Heal Your Life*. The book's basic premise is that we create our own realities and that there is an emotional cause to all diseases. Inside that book, Hay lays out a grid that describes every possible disease, or at least variations of those diseases, and their emotional contributors.

In the case of what I had, colorectal cancer, the primary causes lie in storing up emotions, not letting them go, but also harboring rage and anger. I will tell you with absolute certainty that that's a perfect description of me as a young man. I've spent a lot of time and energy angry and frustrated with someone or something, and I've carried that around with me. I believe it ultimately manifested as a disease.

Most doctors and scientists will all agree that cancer, and disease, for that matter, is caused by several different contributing factors that may include your environment, diet, lifestyle, exercise or lack thereof, and genetic predisposition. Most science professionals that I talk to, who seem reasonably sane, also believe there is an emotional component to disease.

So, don't discount this emotional factor as fuzzy bunny stuff. Instead, as uncomfortable as it may make you feel, dare to give it a chance. Dare to explore the "why" beyond your cancer by delving into your emotional realms. And know that scientists are finding more and more evidence for this connection too.

My Why

So why did you get cancer? Why does anyone get it? You'll get several different responses when you read, watch, or listen to the interviews I do with the survivors at the end of this book.

For me, there were several factors at play. My genetic pre-dispositions: according to my genetic testing, I am 1.4 times more likely to get colorectal cancer than the average person. There were environmental factors: as a child of the '60s and '70s when environmental concerns weren't very high, I essentially spent my formative years playing in toxic waste. I grew up next to fields doused in herbicides and pesticides. I swam in polluted streams and rivers.

Next there's my decades of non-cancer-discouraging eating. I ate lots of bad food and never knew the sources or quality. I drank a lot more than I should have, which harms the immune system. Stress depletes the immune system, and I was a non-stop entrepreneurial stress machine. Consequently, I overtaxed my adrenals for 30+ years. As just mentioned, unhealthy emotions also make a person more susceptible to cancer: I'd been holding onto lots of anger, rage, and unhealthy emotions since I was a kid. Did I mention my years of lack of adequate sleep?

The net result of all this: a toxic time bomb just waiting to go off. As I often say, "It's not what you do once in awhile, it's what you do every day that gets you," I regularly practiced the behavior of cancer cultivation. Anything that constantly causes inflammation, stress, and lowers the immune system is going to catch up with you eventually.

As for the second part of the question, "And does it matter why anyway?" hopefully you can agree that the answer is a resounding YES. After I determined all the factors that could have played a part in me getting cancer, I took a good hard look at everything that I could change for the better. I wanted to do everything in my power to increase the likelihood that my family and I wouldn't have to endure the disease again anytime soon.

Sure, I can't change my genetic predisposition or my childhood encounters with pollution, but I sure as heck can change my diet, my sleep, my tendency to anger, and my stress levels. Yes, it takes a tremendous amount of work and determination to make real changes in these areas, but surviving cancer gives you a second spring. It's up to you to harness that gift, so you can live healthier and happier.

Custodian's Mindset

Just as emotional factors contribute to getting cancer, they also significantly contribute to whether and how a you recover. The fact that so many of the answers the nurses and doctors gave to my question "How can you tell if someone is going to survive or die?" involve emotions, it shouldn't be surprising that the mindset you adopt plays a critical role in your healing.

Aware that my attitude and emotions were going to play a huge role in me surviving (or not), I developed a particular mindset to keep myself in a kind and compassionate state of mind. In case you find it a little odd or "out there," I want to introduce it to you with a little context. Here goes.

Do you remember the movie *Avatar*? In it, a human actor inhabits a genetically-created alien through a form of electronic telepresence. Imagine being able to take over another person's body and look through their eyes and hear, feel, and touch what they experience. Essentially that is the point of view I adopted that allowed me to heal faster because I could disassociate myself from the pain and trauma that was taking place, for nearly a year, in this body that I was inhabiting (so to speak). I call this the custodian's mindset. Here's how it worked.

I didn't say or think "I have cancer." Instead, my dialogue was "My body has cancer." It's my opinion that your body is a vehicle. Your body *is not you.* Think of your body as a perfect car, a perfect vehicle given to you by your Creator. You get to take care of and ride around in this vehicle for about 80 years, statistically speaking. It enables you to experience all the wonders and joys of living a beautiful life. It enables you to experience incredible opportunities and to be creative by actually creating life through it, experiencing the joy of being a parent.

But to associate and call that body "you," I think doesn't serve the beautiful soul that you are. Plus, it makes facing cancer more difficult.

Another key aspect of this custodian's mindset was that in my mind's eye, I took myself out of my vehicle (my body) and watched it (my body) as if it were an actor in a movie. To put it another way: as I was experiencing everything firsthand, I tried to view myself and the experience as if from the outside, as if through the lens of a camera. In this way I became a nonjudgmental observer of the experience and shared as much compassion and love as I possibly could for that body, that beautiful vehicle. Ultimately, I thought of myself as a caretaker for that beautiful body. By taking on this custodian's mindset, I managed to cultivate deeply loving emotions over the course of a very horrendous experience.

By giving my body immense forgiveness, empathy, and compassion, *cancer became an opportunity to change my life forever*. It forced me to change the way I think and become a better person in a positive way. Another benefit of seizing this opportunity and adopting the custodian's mindset was that it allowed me to sidestep the trap of doubt, anger, and negativity, which many doctors and nurses told me were common in people who would lose the battle to cancer.

Without exception, now that I have had the opportunity to live cancer-free for five years, I believe that the custodian's mindset is the secret to my survival. When I share it with other people who have recently learned they have cancer, it seems to resonate.

As an observer of your "actor," give your body forgiveness, empathy, and compassion, and that will help the healing process. Emotions matter. How you manage your emotions likely factors into getting cancer and equally into healing from it.

I'll go so far as to say the emotions you experience when you inhabit your body directly affect how it performs, just like giving plants sunshine helps them grow. Your body will perform better and live longer when you FEEL positive emotions. This is why repeating incantations, prayers, and affirmations are emotional energy amplifiers. It's fertilizer for healing, growth, and abundance.

Up next: equipping yourself with the most accurate and relevant options depends on your ability to ask questions. In the next chapter I share my strategy for effective questioning, whether that's to doctors, medical staff, or other survivors. Knowledge is power in this quest to survive cancer.

Five Questions to Extract the Truth from Your Doctors

An expert knows all the right answers—if you ask the right questions.

—Levi Strauss

Another major contributor to my survival was the kind of questions I asked, who I ask them to, and the order that I ask them in.

In my opinion, the more questions you ask, the higher your chances of survival. Think of it like this: the more questions you ask and the more interest you share in your disease and healing, then the more attention and interest the doctors and staff will give you.

This may sound offensive to some people, but if you give your doctors more intellectual stimulation, they'll give you more attention and focus. You are, in effect, an entertainer or actor. The more interesting and interested you are, then the better your care will be. Just think about it for a few moments: what gets and keeps your attention? Answer: whatever's *not* boring.

The Big 5

We'll start with the 5-question process I employed to gather eye-opening information that doctors otherwise probably would not have revealed. It uses several levels of powerful psychology that forces the doctors or nurses to become more emotionally connected and attached to you (think: humanization) and to disassociate themselves in a way that will cause them to be more honest and open with you.

Something to take into account is that I made my decisions based upon the numbers, the statistics, the odds. Also, I had a driving, guiding goal: to survive long enough so that my young son would have a father until he was at least 18. What this means then is that I was willing to exchange longevity for short-term quality of life, and I wanted to take on any treatments to achieve this goal.

So, when I asked doctors the following series of 5 questions, it was to move them past their robotic, by-the-book responses and get to their from-the-heart, honest-to-God opinions on treatments that would help me achieve this one goal. And that's why I needed a lengthy series of questions—to carefully push them along to this place of greater openness.

#1—Spill It

In speaking to your doctor, start by prompting them to just say what they have to say. For me, that went like this: "Hey doc, I know you need to tell me whatever you need to tell me, so just go ahead and do it."

At that point, the doctor would say, for example, "You have stage 3 colorectal cancer, and here's what I suggest and recommend you do." From there, they'd give a recommendation of surgery and most likely chemotherapy, and then optionally it was radiation. But I wanted to know more than this—I wanted to know what they really, truly recommended in their heart of hearts.

#2—As Your Spouse

My next question: "What would you recommend if I were your spouse?" To this question, the doctor would give me an answer that typically was pretty much the same as what they already recommended.

#3—As Your Child

Question number three: "What would you say or do if I were your child?" Here, you might get a slightly different point of view because the doctor is likely to take into account longevity, where the cancer is, the types of treatments available, and how they may affect the short- or long-term prognosis. So, really good information can emerge from this question.

#4—As You

"What would you do if you were me?" was my fourth question. Again, the doctor may take a different approach. It could be that their strategy may vary when it comes to themselves, depending on their own sense of risk.

#5—Disassociate: The South Pacific Scenario

The final question is the one that yields the most significant information. But the thing to remember is it only works when you ask the other questions first. If you skip the first questions and just ask the final, you won't learn anything significant because there isn't an opportunity to humanize and connect before disassociating. There is a method to this madness—and it's based on complex human behavior and emotions!

The final question goes like this: "Pretend for a moment that someone just like you with your experience, knowledge, wisdom, and expertise is on vacation on an island somewhere in the South Pacific. Pretend you sit down at a bar for a refreshing drink. Another person walks in and sits down next to you. You two start talking while enjoying fine adult beverages together. It's a perfect moment in the perfect ocean air while the sun sets. You and that other person have a great connection—and that's when the second person announces they have the same diagnosis and prognosis as me. What would that doctor say to this person? What recommendations or advice would that doctor probably give?"

At that point, the doctor's face always changes. They smile, look at me, and open up. Finally, I get the whole truth, unedited and unrestrained. Most of the time, the doctor became an actor in the movie I just set up for them, and they're ready to "play along." Let me share a real-life example that happened to me.

When I was investigating getting radiation treatments, I went through these series of questions with a doctor. In response to the final question, the doctor, assuming the identity of the "actor doctor" at that island bar several thousand miles away, answered: "The doctor on the island heard that the new radiation oncologist at this hospital has been having some problems with the calibration of the equipment, so there could be some unnecessary risk. If it were him, he'd go somewhere else. That doctor heard there have been two reports of internal burning due to overexposure."

I can promise you that without asking the right questions the right way, I wouldn't have extracted that information from anyone at a hospital. To this day, I believe I made a very good decision to go to a different hospital to have my radiation done. It probably prevented what could have been short-term or even permanent damage.

The important takeaway: when you ask a variety of questions and you give the doctor an opportunity to disassociate themselves and speak frankly, you can actually get really good information that may save your life, increase the probability of you surviving, or at a minimum, reduce some long-term risks or damage.

In case you aren't aware, most doctors and hospital staff are expressly told not to refer their patients outside of the network. In fact, they must actively push patients to stay in the network. Otherwise, the hospital loses money. The series of questions shows the doctor your persistence and gives the doctor building opportunities to answer frankly without implicating themselves.

Second Opinions

As already mentioned, I got 11 second opinions before I decided what I was going to do. I used the 5-question process each time when garnering a second opinion.

As far as those second opinions go, I had the good fortune of being able to speak to incredible doctors at Scripps Hospital in San Diego. I spoke to doctors at the Mayo Clinic. I spoke to some of the finest doctors at Sloan Kettering in New York. I spoke to doctors at MD Anderson in Texas. Finally I decided to get my radiation treatments at Duke University Hospital in North Carolina.

As mentioned I spoke to a variety of integrative doctors as well, including one who regrettably ended up dying of cancer himself.

For the record, my wife used to work with Dr. Deepak Chopra who is known as one of the finest medical minds and who's also known for being an integrative and spiritual teacher. Even he agreed on the prognosis and treatments that I should take.

Ultimately I got an enormous amount of great information and data based upon the quality and quantity of questions that I asked, which is why I urge you to be similarly proactive.

Good Questioning Beyond Just Doctors

After you've spoken to your doctors, asked them a bunch of questions, and followed the 5-question process, it's also important that you gather good information from others, like other medical professionals and survivors.

Here's my process for when I talk to survivors or other professionals. You start by asking, "Who are you and why should I listen to you?" Then you listen. Open up your mind, open up your heart. This isn't a time to get into an argument.

Next ask them what their specialty or experience is, and whether or not they're accredited. It's important because you can clarify exactly what kind of doctor, for example, they are. You may be calling someone "Dr. Johnston" and then learn she has a PhD in medieval literature or is a doctor of chiropractic, for example. That will have a different value than, let's say, a heart transplant surgeon who's gone through an enormous amount of training and a different type of rigor.

Also, you might learn that your doctor doesn't actually specialized in the area that you need help in. For me, a radiation oncologist wasn't specialized enough. It was important to me that I spoke to someone who specifically was a colorectal radiation oncologist. In the end, I chose someone who not only had this specialty but also had 30 years of experience in it.

More Super Helpful Questions

After those 5 questions, I've found the following to be very helpful. These are questions I ask survivors:

- How did you deal with the news?
- What was the first thing that ran through your mind?
- How has your relationship with yourself changed?
- How has your relationship with God or your creator changed?
- How has your relationship with your spouse, child or children, other family members, business, employees, friends, or other people in your life changed?
- What do you wish you would have done now that you've been through it? (Yes, I ask regret questions.)

The following I ask survivors, doctors, or other medical staff:

- What's the best advice you've ever given to someone just like me?
- What's the best advice you've ever received?
- What kind of treatment recommendations do you have?
- I also ask diet questions: what did you eat or do you

recommend I eat? What made you feel bad? Good?

- I ask fitness questions and recovery questions.
- I ask about resources: are there resources, apps, software, systems, tools, foods, supplements, books, or user groups that you recommend?

If you learn how to ask questions like this, you can become an expert on practically any topic in a very short period of time. The point is to ask, speak up, and advocate for yourself, your health, your present, and your future. Don't worry about sounding silly or dumb or about inconveniencing someone.

The more questions you ask, the more you can separate the good information and possibilities from the bad. The more options you give yourself. The more you prove to the experts that you are worth their time and interest as well.

Up next: managing how you communicate and connect with others—from medical staff to close family and friends and to colleagues and acquaintances—is something you need to have a strategy for. That's what the next chapter is about.

Communication Strategies

Love your neighbor, yet don't pull down your hedge.
—Benjamin Franklin

Getting the cancer diagnosis can knock you off your feet. The cancer itself in combination with the treatments will give you levels of fatigue you've never encountered. During this time, connecting with others, whether that be your doctor, your child, or an acquaintance, will suddenly become very demanding. Plain old physically and mentally tough. That's why I've written this chapter: to give you options to more easily manage communication.

Tech to the Rescue

When you are going through the treatments, you are very likely going to be fatigued. It's going to be hard for you to recall information. If you haven't heard of brain fog or chemo brain before, it is very real. You will experience cognitive impairment, and it will be crazy difficult to remember certain facts or keep things in a specific order.

When this happens, communicating in a coherent way, not only with medical staff but also with your close family, becomes problematic. My solution: the audio recorder on my phone. I got into a habit of recording all the important conversations.

An audio recording platform that I highly recommend is something called www.Rev.com. Rev.com not only lets you record conversations, but it also allows you to press a button and have transcripts made of those conversations.

Another utility that is really good if you want to record phone conversations is an app called TapeACall. You press a button, and your phone will record a phone call. That way you have those saved and stored too. Plus, TapeACall offers transcripts of your recorded calls through Rev.com.

Mike's Cancer Communication Rules

It's of utmost importance that you create rules on how you want others to communicate with you regarding your cancer. You might think I'm being over the top, so let me paint a picture on why these rules are peace-of-mind savers.

When you notify a few people that you have cancer, that news is going to travel quickly. Many, many people, possibly hundreds, are going to start calling you, texting you, and emailing you, giving all sorts of unsolicited opinions, solutions, and referrals. They will direct you to talk to a certain person, and they'll even talk to others on your behalf. It's like all these people are under the illusion that you desperately want their advice in the first place.

Already you are feeling fatigued from the cancer itself, from the emotion around the news of the diagnosis, from your treatment strategy (if you've decided it yet). So when all these people are contacting you, thinking they're doing you a favor by giving their opinions, what will happen is that your tiredness and stress will only increase.

While it's unlikely you'll care about their advice, you'll want to acknowledge them and their attempt at showing concern. But, you'll also feel bombarded and just plain tired. Taking on all the contact becomes too much, overwhelming. That's why I urge you to create some rules of communication.

As soon as I was diagnosed and had a plan in mind, I sent out a message to everyone I knew in which I was very specific about the kind of help I wanted and didn't want. In my message, I was careful to explain why I was making the rules: "I'm getting hundreds of messages a day. While I know you have the best of intentions, it's impossible to navigate all of them. I don't have the time or staff members to sort through all the advice."

Next, instead of cutting everyone off and going cold, I laid down rules on how I wanted people to communicate their cancer advice to me.

First, I created a separate email, and I set up a Google phone number. Then I explained that I didn't want to receive any cancer information to my main email address, and I didn't want any phone calls. That's what the special email and phone number were for.

Second, I was very specific on how I wanted any information communicated to me. I didn't want to receive books, pamphlets, or a list of links. Instead, if someone had something to share, I asked them to summarize it in one paragraph, telling what they wanted to send, why it should matter, and how I could use it. I followed that up with, "Then you can provide the links or materials." Notice that I was explicit about *not* wanting any raw links or raw information. I wanted them first to interpret *why* it was valuable.

Here's what happened: my rules cut off 90% of all of the flow. My rules stopped the flow of the useless information, and I only got the good stuff.

Another handy resource for managing the deluge of communications you'll get is a website at (www.CaringBridge.org). Caring Bridge is a service that allows you to set up a free website where people can communicate with you and you can post progress and pictures. It's like an active blog. On it people can post feedback and suggestions, and most importantly, you get to navigate through all of it in one place. That's another solution that could further simplify the communication challenge. However, even with Caring Bridge, I urge you to establish some rules.

Progress Reports

Let me preface this part by stating in no uncertain terms: you're the one in charge of making the rules for how you want to communicate with others about your cancer. Also, you don't owe anyone anything. Cancer is so challenging that sometimes just taking caring of yourself is all you can manage. And that's okay. You don't owe anyone an explanation of what and how you are doing. That's not your responsibility.

For me, it was very important that I communicated on a regular basis with the large group of people beyond my closest circle of family and friends. You see, I have a large group of people—friends, acquaintances, clients, business associates, and customers—that I'd been active with over years. Because I knew these people were interested in what was going on with me and because I didn't want any rumors to get started (that's an additional purpose of this book), it was important to me to send out regular group messages about my progress with cancer.

In these "progress reports" I was able to communicate with everyone and answer all their questions in one place. This ended up being a very powerful strategy. Plus, I didn't have to go through and reply to everyone individually.

Again, the Caring Bridge platform also offers a convenient way to keep your broader audience informed on your progress—*if* that's something you feel inclined to do.

Your Nearest and Dearest

As soon as I found out that I had cancer, my wife was the first to know. From that point on, I didn't make any big decisions without her input. It was important to me that she got involved with everything.

I let all my doctors, family, and friends know how important her input and presence were for me. She was involved in every conversation about diagnosis, treatment, and everything major happening with the business, partnerships, promotions, and transition plans.

Never try to "protect" your spouse—because if you find yourself in a position at some point where things start falling apart and your spouse doesn't know what's going on, it's probably going to be worse. It's not up to you to edit, filter, or determine what someone can or can't handle.

Plus, you're not going to be in a powerful state of mind once the treatments kick in. You won't always be cogent. The term "chemo-brain" exists because it is real. You'll be tired, fatigued, and not feel like yourself. So learn to let go of trying to be a superhuman.

Most likely both your and your spouse's "stories" about who each of you are are outdated and based on all sorts of assumptions and predisposed opinions that are no longer relevant or accurate. Cancer gives you an opportunity to reinvent your relationship and reframe and rewrite your rules of engagement. Take this opportunity to listen, learn, and grow. Weak minds don't survive this process. Both of you need to be strong. This is all stuff I'm going to go into more in later chapters.

Talking to your children about your cancer is not easy or comfortable either, but it's essential that you do it to avoid any misunderstanding on their part. As soon as I knew what was going on, I sat down with my son, Zak, who was 10 at the time, and I let him know that I was sick, that I knew I'd be okay, and that my sickness had nothing to do with him. It was just my body. I reaffirmed that I loved him and that that would never change.

Then I tried to preemptively clarify any confusion he might have down the road. I explained to him that I wouldn't have the same amount of energy to play and spend time with him as I normally did, but that that didn't mean I didn't love him. I explained the lack of energy was temporary and wasn't going to last forever. I explained that feeling so tired was actually normal. The medicine would make me tired, but eventually it would heal me.

Believe me, when this tiredness showed up there were times that were so hard for both me and my son. We live next to the ocean in San Diego, and one of my son's favorite things to do is to swim in the ocean. It was a normal thing for Zak to ask me, "Daddy, can you go swimming with me?"

When you are going through chemotherapy, it is not uncommon to have neuropathy and to be extremely temperature sensitive. I remembering feeling absolutely miserable. I had no energy. Just opening the refrigerator door felt like someone was smacking my face with a bag of broken glass.

So when Zak asked me to go swimming with him, I knew that just putting my toe into the ocean would feel like I was standing on broken glass or hot flowing lava because my temperature sense had completely changed. Hot was cold and cold was hot. It hurt. It was horrible.

I let Zak know that there needed to be other ways that we could spend time together. Because I was so clear that the cancer had nothing to do with me loving him, he was fine with that.

No matter the age of your children, I strongly encourage you to talk to them about your cancer, let them in on how you'll be feeling during your treatments (in an age-appropriate way, of course), and assure them that you love them. They'll be scared, concerned, and confused, so these kinds of conversations are essential. Because this is such an important issue, I'm dedicating a whole chapter to it as well.

If you are wondering about communicating with your closest friends and family, for me, even with them I only let a select few know at first. I wanted to make sure that I, personally, was clear on exactly what was going to happen and what my treatment plan was before I got into long complicated conversations with the people in my inner circle.

Later, once I'd made these plans, I used the "progress reports" that I described earlier to keep both my inner and largest circle informed on where I was at.

To repeat, it isn't your responsibility to keep anyone and everyone updated on how you are going with cancer. You are in charge of how or whether you want to inform others. For me, it worked to set very clear communication guidelines and to send regular progress reports.

Up next: we continue the discussion of communication, more specifically—how to stay connected and relevant to your business base while facing cancer.

Marketing While You're Away

The less you open your heart to others, the more your heart suffers.

—Deepak Chopra

Here's one of the biggest fears I had at that time period: I was afraid that I would announce to my customers that I had cancer and I was sick, and then—they would abandon me. After that, I wouldn't be able to take care of my family. I would appear weak and fragile.

If you are an entrepreneur, as I am, I bet you can relate to this massive fear.

Now, for the reality: when I reached out and told my customers and business associates that I had cancer, the amount of love and positive response was absolutely overwhelming. I quickly realized that I had nothing to be afraid of. But, it didn't stop there.

In this chapter I share the marketing I did to keep my business intact and to keep my customers, business associates, and large audience involved while I was removed from the business, facing the cancer. Because all of this involves communication, you can expect this chapter to build off the previous one.

Client Kinship

Let's start with what I do. For 15+ years, I've been helping people start and run their own entrepreneurial businesses, training and teaching them online. At one point, I had two software companies, well over 40,000 customers over those companies' histories, and earned tens of millions of dollars online.

My customers, business associates, and I tend to feel a connection. This feeling of kinship is something my business partners and I find important to foster with our customers. Our customers look to me as a source of impact, income, lifestyle and vision. Many of them fed their families as result of the tools and the resources that my businesses provided them.

Because of this closeness, I knew that simply telling them I had cancer and then taking time away wasn't for me. To stay relevant to them—and more importantly, for me to feel them rallying for me—I wanted to keep them involved with my journey (or battle) as I progressed through it. That's where the "progress reports" that I described in the previous chapter came in.

Starring Michael Koenigs as "Man Battling Cancer"

When I first informed my large business base that I had cancer, I didn't just relate the diagnosis. For me, it was important that I mustered the courage and confidence to say that I felt absolutely certain that I was going to survive.

After that, I kept them involved through the regular progress reports I sent out. Here's the thing about those progress reports that made them really work for me. They came in the form of emails *and* videos.

I did everything I could to create a narrative, a "movie" about my experience, one that I personally would find interesting, moving, and informative and that my clients and customers would want to watch and read too. This isn't to say that I created something that wasn't real; it was absolutely authentic and as real as possible. It was brutally honest, and that's why it was so compelling.

Remember earlier when I explained the custodian's mindset? Quick recap: it's the mindset I adopted where I came to see my body as this vehicle that I was taking caring of. I learned to observe my body as if it were an actor in a movie, and I was the audience simply watching. This mindset allowed me greater peace of mind and courage. It allowed me to experience less frustration and anger as well.

The narrative I presented through these emails and videos helped me to embrace this powerful mindset even more. At the same time, it allowed my large circle of clients, business associates, and friends to become involved and sympathetic participants as well.

Another benefit of making these movies and sending out the emails is that like any kind of publicity, if you aren't the one making the news, then someone else will do it for you, for better or worse. The last thing you need or want are rumors to begin. I thought long and hard about what kind of rumors could get started and what kind of fears or concerns might occur that could run out of control and cause damage to the business and to my employees as well. As a result, I decided it was essential that I was the one producing the news around my cancer journey, not anyone else.

Another thing I did that turned out to be one of the best decisions of my life is I began writing a book while I was going through the last phases of treatment. I used that book as a mechanism for communicating to my audience that it was possible to make a difference and share a message even while undergoing tough cancer treatments.

To be completely transparent, that book ended up becoming the framework for a course that guides business owners on how to write books. That has since turned into a multimillion-dollar franchise called Publish and Profit.

Getting back to what is relevant for you and how to go about marketing while facing cancer: just know that like in any good business environment, you have to know who your market is and what the message needs to be. The message that you have for your immediate friends and family will be very different than that for your spouse or children or that for your employees, clients, and customers.

With that in mind, I thought long and hard about what my various audience's concerns were and what information about my cancer journey would be important to them to know. Without a lot of work I was able to create short videos and the appropriate messaging that made the most sense for the particular audience at hand.

My Marketing Shortcuts

These shortcuts may have come about because I really needed them from the extreme fatigue I was suffering during my time battling cancer, but many are so good I use them to this day.

In the previous chapter I told you about Rev.com. I learned to use this service not only to record and get transcribed important conversations with doctors, but also to create business-related content. I'm even using it to write this very book.

I was very fortunate that a very good friend offered me business support the moment I announced that I had cancer. His name is Ed Rush, and he is a very smart and capable copywriter and business associate. We were friends and had participated in a Mastermind group together.

Ed ended up becoming my voice and my number one copywriter and marketer. He was not only able to write in my voice while I was away and being treated, but my business actually started making more money while I was gone. What an eye-opening lesson! As hard-driving entrepreneurs, we believe we are essential for all aspects of our business, but sometimes it's good for us to disappear for a while, so our employees and team can self-organize.

The bottom line and the net result: Ed Rush became my voice. I had a story, a plan, and a strategy for how to communicate with my various channels: my clients, customers, vendors, employees, and family members. I gave them what they needed to be comfortable. Through the narratives I crafted in my emails and videos, I made the experience interesting, dynamic, and exciting, so they felt like they had a front-row seat at a movie that was for them.

I want to acknowledge that what I'm describing may sound commercial to you, but it taught me an incredibly valuable lesson about empathy and compassion. To this day I believe this is one of the most important lessons I've ever received in my business and personal life: when you allow others into the intimate heartbreaks and triumphs you experience, so they can really feel what you are going through, they will *not* respond with rejection, mockery, disinterest, or cynicism. In fact, they will embrace you with full-on empathy and compassion.

I call this "emotional amplitude." If an actor takes you on a journey with big highs and low lows, the audience will create a much stronger bond with the actor very quickly. Emotions are like music—when there's more volume and variability, there is generally more impact.

I'll add too that sharing your cancer experience in a full and honest way with others, even when your body is experiencing an enormous amount of pain, allows you a truly remarkable gift of tremendous compassion and empathy. It isn't just your audience who is getting emotionally impacted by your experience. They, in turn, feed and nurture you with their emotional concern and support. It's a win-win.

When I returned back to work after my final treatment, we prepared a new product launch and a special live event that we called a "Celebration of Life Party." As I think about it right now and share it with you, I'm getting very choked up recalling the incredible amount of compassion and empathy my customers and audience shared with me.

At this "Celebration of Life Party" product launch, so many people showed up and embraced me. It ended up being incredibly successful, generating millions of dollars in revenue. It is a perfect example of how no matter how bad you think things might get or how they actually might be, there are plenty of people who are there to support you and provide for you when you least expect it—especially when you take them with you on your rocky journey.

To be clear: I'm *not* suggesting for a moment that you commercialize or profit from your illness. That's NOT the point. All I'm saying is the more transparent and vulnerable you are, the more support and care you'll receive. To me, the opposing end is playing the victim, making everything about you and being miserable and self-absorbed. Nobody wants to be around that energy, and as I already shared, the nurses and doctors identified that stance as the one that leads to decline and death.

Up next: let's extend this look at business by considering the core team necessary for keeping your business going while you're away.

The People You Need for Your Company's Survival

Great things in business are never done by one person.
They're done by a team of people.

—Steve Jobs

Even though this book is called "Cancerpreneur" and is business-biased, this chapter is simple because teaching you how to run a business isn't my goal. You already know how to do that. The secret to surviving and thriving has to do more with psychology, in terms of the questions you ask and decisions you make that are outside of the business itself.

You're going to get the most business value by reading, listening to, or watching the doctor and survivor interviews, at the end of this book, and on the site www.Cancerpreneur.com.

Even still, there's a few aspects of your business that I want to address, primarily the people you need for your company's survival when you're away battling cancer. You're going to need a core team of people that you can trust to keep the business vibrant.

Based on my own experience and in speaking to other entrepreneurs and business owners who've gone through similar challenges, here's the team that I recommend in order of value:

- a personal or executive assistant
- someone in operations
- someone in marketing and communications
- someone in sales
- someone in accounting, if possible

Of course, all this depends on the size of your business, the revenue that you generate, and how dependent your organization is on you being there all the time. The smaller you are, the more challenging this can be, but never underestimate your team's ability to adapt and contribute when you give them the opportunity to do so.

Let me explain my thinking about the importance of the given team members.

A Personal Assistant

I would say that, hands down, having a really good personal assistant or executive assistant will improve your life a thousand-fold. That's the first person you need on your core team.

In my case, my assistant, Laurie Hull, who has now worked with me for 11 years, has been instrumental, an absolutely powerful advocate who's been imperative to my business.

Laurie knows practically everything about me: my calendar, my schedule, all of my personal information. She can make travel arrangements and knows how to coordinate with all my other team members. She's also responsible for my customer support and a lot of the details that revolve around the events that I do.

Laurie is indispensable. And when you are going through cancer, your assistant who was already indispensable will only become even more so.

When you watch or listen to the bonus videos with other survivors, you'll learn how they too depended on their assistants.

Operations

The key to your business continuing to generate money while you are dealing with life and death lies in you already having a team in place that can run everything without you—*before* you need them to.

In my case, before cancer crossed my radar, I had

Gene Naftulyev, a business turnaround specialist, come in and help me increase the profitability of my business. He replaced "people" with "processes" and helped to take me as much out of the decision-making loop as possible, so I could focus on big-picture items. He made it so I could work *on* the business rather than *in* it.

By doing this before my cancer, later when I was dealing with cancer, Gene was able to keep the company running with my good friend Ed Rush who focused on the marketing.

During the weeks where I had to devote all of my time and limited energy on myself, I still shot some videos and took phone calls with partners and affiliates. However, for the most part, because of its operational efficiency, my company was not only able to carry on doing business, but actually managed to return a higher profit at the end of the year than the previous year—all while I was dealing with cancer. If there's one thing I'd recommend, no matter what takes you away from your business, that's have a trusted, efficient operations team in place—before you ever need them.

Setting up operational efficiency requires that you systemize and document what you and your team do on a regular basis. Every single activity must have a "standard operating procedure" or SOP. We make short videos that a new person can watch to learn how a particular task is handled. When I was sick, I made short videos and sent then to my team, so I didn't have to work around their schedule.

Marketing and Communications

In the previous chapter, I described how key it was for me to keep my marketing and communications going. To summarize, my personal connection with my large base was an essential element in the success of my business, so it would've been unwise for me to go radio silent for a whole year. I was beyond lucky to have Ed Rush in charge of this arena. I put all my faith in him to communicate in my voice for me and take on the marketing, and his competence and wisdom exceeded my lofty expectations and needs.

For Ed to be able to completely fill his role, he had to be able to speak and write in my voice and be comfortable with the systems my business used: InfusionSoft for our CRM, Kajabi for delivering membership sites, ClickFunnels for building sales pages, a product called WebinarJam for automating sales webinars, and Zoom Meetings for hosting meetings and doing coaching. And, of course, he was.

For your cash flow to continue while you're away, you'll need someone like Ed will also follow a general marketing schedule. That way you'll at least be able to stay relevant to your business associates and customers, which will keep the money machine rolling.

Having a good support team makes a big difference. In my case, I had customer service and customer support. If I would have had to shrink the company down considerably, my personal assistant would have been able to fill in the gaps—and many times she did.

Sales

Then there's sales. Again, we were able to deal with that. In a pinch, my marketing team, support team, and even my assistant could manage incoming and outgoing sales calls. The point is that you're always looking for some ways to keep that income and revenue coming in.

Finances

Finally, having someone either full- or part-time who can manage accounting issues is super valuable.

We became ruthless with eliminating expenses, finding waste, and simplifying the business while I was away.

That's what made the biggest difference. Our profits increased even though our revenues decreased.

Interns

One of the things that happened while I was away is my operations team started bringing interns into the business. The interns would work for minimum wage or in some cases actually volunteer. That made a huge impact on getting small things done and wound up swinging big doors.

This was another way we were able to reduce our internal costs considerably while maintaining productivity and profitability.

An Active Wellspring in Dry Times

Having some source of income while you are facing cancer is out-of-the-universe helpful.

When I got diagnosed with cancer, my business was going through some significant turmoil. Due to a substantial change in market behavior it was in decline. Much of our marketing and sales weren't effective, and we were carrying around an enormous amount of overhead.

My operations team quickly started to surgically eliminate an enormous amount of waste and overspending. In addition to this, what saved the business was the fact that we had some subscription income. While I was away, I was able to think about and invent some new products, portions of which could be created without my direct involvement.

I think what is important to take into account, and you will experience this when you read the Hal Elrod interview, is the possibility of passive income. Hal was fortunate enough to have written a book that brought in tens of thousands of dollars in income per month, and it actively promoted his events and coaching. So when he was facing cancer, this passive income benefitted him and his family not just financially and physically (in that he did not have to actively solicit it) but also emotionally. He had so much to worry and stress about—because that's what happens with cancer, it's scary—but his money worries were minimal.

It is essential for us, as entrepreneurs, to always be on the lookout for ways to create income that doesn't directly require us to be actively working it. This way we can gain some level of leverage in difficult times. Without that, we have very little to depend on.

I can selfishly say, if you're interested in learning how to write a book or create a product, both effective passive income generators, you should definitely visit one of my websites to learn more about how you can do this, even while you are sick.

Up next: just like a core team of only the most competent and trustworthy individuals is essential for your business to survive, there are some core dietary guidelines you must follow to keep your vulnerable body at its healthiest.

Daily Medicine: Diet

Let food be thy medicine and medicine be thy food.
—Hippocrates

Food is so important, and it's typically very misunderstood. A tremendous number of doctors are horribly incompetent when it comes to food and diet. In fact, most oncologists tell their patients that it doesn't matter what you eat, and it won't affect anything. I believe this advice is a horrible injustice and, at some point, will be considered a crime. It will be treated the same way as someone smoking cigarettes in an operating room.

The key things that I want to cover in this chapter are how to listen to your body, who to listen to, what foods to get rid of, and what foods to eat. I am going to make some recommendations and suggestions on what I've eaten and how I've changed my diet and body as well.

Hear That?

The most important lesson, one that I didn't do while I was going through treatment, is to listen to your body.

I now know how to listen to my body. When I put some food in my mouth and start chewing it, I pay very close attention to how my body reacts and how I feel. If I can tell that there is a slight reaction, for example, if my nose itches, I get scratchy, or I can feel my stomach start to change or churn a little bit, I spit out the food. These slight reactions are my body's way of warning me that the food is going to cause inflammation.

A body that is inflamed is more vulnerable to disease. It means your immune system is being overstressed. Especially when you are facing cancer, inflammation is something you want to avoid.

In my case, I was diagnosed with stage 3a colorectal cancer. I underwent surgery, chemotherapy, and radiation treatment. The type of surgery I had involved something called resectioning: they cut out my entire sigmoid colon, a third of my rectum, and stapled me back together. The result: it took a long time for my body to start processing food. On top of that, due to the nature of being on antibiotics and having very low white blood cell counts, it took a long time for my stomach and bowels to start working again as well.

If you are receiving chemotherapy of any sort, your stomach flora is going to be severely damaged. This flora contributes to your body's ability to absorb nutrients, so when it gets killed or damaged, the energy your body receives from ingested nutrients dramatically decreases. Consequently, your rate of healing slows or grinds to a halt, which is the last thing you want. You need a constant supply of probiotic-rich foods or supplements to replace that damaged flora.

Because your body's ability to take in nutrients is already so compromised, it should motivate you to seek out the most nutrient-rich foods and totally avoid the nutrient-depleting ones. If you pay careful attention to your body, as I described in the start of this section, it will even tell you if the food you are eating is going to help or hurt it. But you must learn to listen—and that takes practice.

Adios to the Biggest Evils

From my time spent with people in nutrition, fitness, and health care and from working with many integrative doctors, I am a passionate believer in the importance of diet. I cannot urge you enough to follow a very specific diet (which I'll soon describe) and cut out what the acclaimed nutritionist J. J. Virgin calls the "biggest evils." Why? Because not all calories are created equal; some heal and some hurt. The "biggest evils" are (obviously) the ones that hurt us.

It is essential that you get rid of the most "evil" food out there: refined sugar. Scientists, nutritionists, and medical professionals who have a clue agree that refined sugar is one of the most toxic substances that you can put in your body, yet hospitals are still serving sugar in soft drinks and juices on a regular basis. To me, that's the same as serving poison.

Sugar will eventually damage your body or cause diseases that can kill you. There's hard scientific evidence to show that sugar is not only highly addictive, but cancer cells feed on it. As an old saying goes, don't piss in your gas tank. Your car won't run well.

After sugar, the "biggest evils" to remove from your diet, in order, are dairy, wheat, soy, corn, and for many people, peanuts and eggs, all of which can be very inflammatory.

It goes without saying that you do not want to drink alcohol at all while you are undergoing treatment. I have to admit that I did drink some wine occasionally while I was undergoing treatment, and I knew at the time that it was hurtful and harmful.

I'm not suggesting that you can't treat yourself every once in awhile with something. Before you put anything negative or bad in your stomach, drink a big glass of water first and see if that takes some of the desire away.

Next, get rid of all processed foods. If it is white, in a bag, a box, or a can, it probably isn't good for you and is going to do more damage than good.

Key things to make certain that you keep out of your diet are sugar (can't repeat this enough), nearly all protein bars (which are mostly sugar), fruit juices, and absolutely, positively no soda. Most nutritionists who know anything agree that diet soda is just as unhealthy as sugar-based soda. My advice: drink only water, especially when you are being treated.

Again, a lot of medical doctors without a nutrition background will tell you some sort of nonsense along the lines of "Get any kind of calories inside your body as you can. It's all good." I believe that is, again, a point of view that will soon be viewed as being as irresponsible as telling someone it's okay to smoke two packs of cigarettes a day.

Anticancer Eating

Many people seeking positive and anti-cancerous eating look to the Virgin Diet, popularized by my friend J.J. Virgin, the well-known celebrity nutrition expert, and also by my friend, Dave Asprey, from Bulletproof Coffee. *To be totally transparent, I am an early-stage investor in Bulletproof, the company Dave founded, but what I'm about to say about diet has nothing to do with this affiliation.*

Along with the Virgin Diet I recommend researching a paleo or ketogenic diet. These diets change your body's focus away from burning sugar to burning fat.

Stay away from carbs—especially processed carbs. Anything that comes in a bag, box, or can is probably a processed or simple carb. The body simply will turn it into sugar. Cancer likes sugar.

There are a lot of people who believe that a pure vegan diet is anti-cancerous. This could be true as long as the vegan diet isn't based on fructose or sugar. Unfortunately, a lot of vegans and vegetarians eat food that is high in sugar or has wheat, soy, corn, or peanuts in it. Wheat, soy, corn, and peanuts are known to have very strong inflammatory responses inside the human body. As already explained, a body that is inflamed is subject to disease. It means your immune system is being overstressed, and that has a negative effect on you.

What diet do I recommend? I'll first begin by saying I'm not a nutritionist. I'm not a doctor, and I don't play one on TV or the Internet. The diet that I've found that's had the most positive response on me, and I have the blood tests to back it up, is a keto-style diet.

Eat high-quality protein. If you eat fish, make sure the fish is young. That's because older fish often have higher amounts of heavy metal poisoning, like mercury, in them. Tuna, for example, is an older fish. You want to eat fish that is two years old or younger, like salmon, sole, or freshwater fish.

Through my DNA tests, I learned that "bloody red" meats increase my chances of colon cancer recurrence, so I don't eat those anymore. That means no more lamb, beef, deer, elk, etc. Instead, I eat high-quality organic chicken and pork. I'm also told to avoid any meats that are charred.

Make sure you consume high-quality fats, like that from avocados. You can also consider adding MCT, or Brain Octane Oil, from Bulletproof Labs. (Again, I am an early-stage investor in Bulletproof, but you can find other products that have the same components in them.)

Eat lots of steamed veggies.

Raw foods are generally very difficult for the body to digest, and this is one of the reasons why eating a raw food vegan diet may not be ideal, depending on the state and strength of your digestive system. The rule of thumb is if you are gassy or getting gas, you want to reduce or eliminate the amount of raw foods in your diet. You don't want your body to work harder than it needs to.

Most dieticians and nutritionists agree that when you combine high-quality protein and high-quality fats, and you eat those before you succumb to eating sugar, you'll feel full.

No matter what some doctors will tell you, when you stick to simple diets that are anti-inflammatory, you are going to feel better and heal faster too.

Up next: I discuss the effects of cancer on your marriage and how, with courage on both your parts, you can turn the sickness into an opportunity for greater unity.

Your Marriage

Through my research, I found that vulnerability is the glue that holds relationships together. It's the magic sauce.

—Brene Brown

When I was diagnosed, my wife, Vivian, stood by me. She became my advocate. She put herself and her own needs and interests aside, as I went through the grueling process.

When I look at my years before cancer, I now see I was far too busy for far too long. I wasn't involved like a good spouse or father could or should be. I was an overly busy, overly enthusiastic, hard-driving entrepreneur who was most afraid of going broke, losing my status, and not being top in my game. I was always working for more, more, more, instead of focusing on what I already had and being grateful for that.

Cancer offers a unique opportunity to reassess and realign your values. If you look at things through courageous eyes, the quality of your marriage can actually increase and improve during this trying time. Here's how it happened for me.

The Big C and S-E-X

It's an understatement to say that while you go through treatments that include surgery, chemotherapy, and radiation, your sex drive is reduced. As I already shared, I was horribly afraid that I would be permanently damaged in terms of sex. It's not uncommon for someone with colorectal cancer to wake up with no sex drive at all and some kind of irreversible damage or nerve damage caused by surgery, complications from surgery, or radiation.

In that sense, it wasn't different for me. Everything that involved any kind of sexual contact flat out hurt. It was a burning sensation that was very unpleasant, which certainly doesn't translate into a lot of fulfillment or interest for you or your partner. For me, this was actually a positive. Let me explain.

In nearly all of my past relationships I put an enormous amount of value and pressure on my partner for sex. Sex every day was my goal. I also put a lot of pressure on myself to perform.

Cancer offered me a unique and beautiful opportunity to focus on my relationship with my wife outside of sex. In this way cancer became the cure for my negative belief system and behavior in which I equated intimacy, love, and sex together. I learned very rapidly that intimacy and love were not the same thing as sex, and vice versa. This was a huge insight that has vastly improved my marriage.

Hoffman and Healing

The number one thing that made the biggest difference in my marriage was a weeklong course I participated in that offered emotional and behavioral healing treatments. After I finished my treatment, which was approximately one year from the time I was diagnosed, I took a course called the Hoffman Process. (You can learn more about this remarkable program by visiting the resource section in this book or going to the website, www.HoffmanInstitute.org).

Through this course I finally learned how to fully and completely forgive myself, come to terms with my past, and to let go of lots of old stories and trauma that I had carried with me for decades that I believe contributed to the emotional cause of my cancer. Doing this intense therapeutic self-work helped me to be more available, connected, and supportive to my wife in our continuing partnership.

For You and Your Spouse

What are my recommendations for your marriage and how to get through the process? I think the first and most important thing is that you manage expectations. Be sure that your partner understands that you are going to be physically, mentally, and emotionally unavailable part of the time and that you are going to drift in and out of being accessible and cogent. Just like with your children and the rest of your business, what you're going through has absolutely nothing to do with your spouse, meaning your inaccessibility is not personal.

Much like going through a home remodel, the illness can cause irreparable harm to a marriage if the two of you aren't committed to communicating and being compassionate and empathic. To help you and your spouse manage expectations and make sure you stay connected, therapy can be a great help. Consider beginning therapy as quickly as possible and stick to a regular schedule so that each of you can communicate what you're experiencing in a safe environment.

The honest truth is, it's going to be harder on your spouse than it is for you because they will be watching you go through pain and anguish and dealing with people who neither of you know and taking advice without understanding what is really wrong and what the possibilities and probabilities for permanent damage are.

My advice to all non-sick spouses is, never make this disease or the treatment about you. Instead, just be present and do everything you can to participate in the healing process for your sick spouse. If you have children, focus on creating an opportunity for your partner to spend high-quality and meaningful time with the children without taxing their immune system too much.

In summary my advice for both parties is to manage your expectations and practice patience, empathy, and compassion. Get regular therapy if you think that will facilitate a better connection. Once you've gone through treatment, consider enrolling in the Hoffman Process because it will profoundly improve the quality of your relationship with your spouse and with yourself. It will transform who you are, so you can fully integrate the benefits of going through the cancer experience.

Up next: we return to your relationship with your children during this time of cancer.

Cancer and Your Kids

It is easier to build strong children than to repair broken men.

—Frederick Douglass

There are some important considerations to take into account when it comes to your cancer and your children: their sense of safety and their understanding of your changing body.

Their Sense of Safety

When you tell your children that you have cancer, make sure you are providing an environment where they are able to safely communicate how they feel, what they're fearing, and what they're experiencing. Try to allow them to express.

At the same time, it is vitally important that you give your children hope and confidence so that they experience a minimum amount of trauma.

Remember, there's a lot of unknowns going on, both for you and your family. Perhaps your survival is at question and that can be incredibly traumatic for any child. The lack of knowledge, inability to predict what will happen next, lack of control—all those unknowns are what can cause long-term damage if not handled properly. Once again, I believe it is extremely valuable that you get a good therapist to work with you and your family.

Another aspect to your children's sense of safety involves them not ever thinking that your cancer is their fault. When you are first diagnosed, it is essential that you remind your children that your cancer has nothing to do with them, that they're not at fault, and that you love them no matter what. This is when it is important to talk to them about how you'll be changing as well.

Your Changing Body

To help them feel safe and reduce their trauma, you'll have to regularly talk to them about your changing body. Let your children know that there will be times when you are too weak from the medicine, too tired or fatigued, or may even have a bad attitude, but it has nothing to do with them. It's just that your body's really tired, and you might not have control over your emotions.

An interesting but relevant metaphor is the whole notion of being "hangry." That's when you're hungry and angry at the same time. If you can relate that to your children and remind them of a time that they felt frustrated and angry only because they hadn't eaten in a long time. Let them know you'll be going through something similar to that.

Again, purposefully articulate that your cancer has absolutely nothing to do with them, that you are there for them, but that you just might not be able to spend as much time with them as you are used to.

Another aspect of the changing body is the fact that there will be certain activities that you won't be capable of doing. Depending on the treatment that you go through, there will be a certain amount of recovery time when you're not able to be as physical as you normally are. With chemotherapy, you'll definitely go through phases where you'll have a lot of fatigue or be indisposed on the toilet on a very regular basis. Or, the byproduct of chemotherapy, which could be mild or severe neuropathy. That's when you lose sensation in your fingers or toes temporarily or get extremely cold-sensitive.

As a parent, I believe it's important that you provide a sense of comfort and hope on a regular basis; that you show courage and confidence and become a bright shining star. As I mentioned earlier a few times now, I thought of the cancer process as a movie, and my body as an actor. (Remember, the custodian's mindset?) I imagined that there were cameras on me at all times, so I wanted to make the cancer experience something that I was proud of, that I'd want to watch again some day. This mindset helped me maintain strength of character for my family and also for myself.

There are going to be times when you're so overwhelmed or you're so tired and fatigued that it's difficult to make good decisions. Sometimes you're overpowered by that. But I was careful to remind myself and my son that it was my body that had the disease and that it wasn't me. I explained that there would be times when I'd lose my hair, I'd lose a lot of weight, or I'd look really sickly, but that it still was me inside this body and that I loved him no matter what.

In summary I think it's important to communicate what you're experiencing in a way that your children understand without putting them in a place where they're fearful. Also, they must always know that you love them, no matter what your body is doing or prevents you from doing.

Up next: speaking of our changing bodies, it's time we talk about working out. The next chapter addresses working out at diagnosis, during treatment, and after treatment.

Exercise and Self-Care

You can't hire someone else to do your push-ups for you.
—Jim Rohn

A lack of exercise affects not only our physical state but our mental state too. Exercising is something positive that we can control, so even after a cancer diagnosis, it is hard to give it up.

After I was diagnosed, I continued my active exercise habits. I thought it would really help my mind and body. I figured it was super important that I keep it up. So, I went outside. I did a lot of running. What ended up happening is that it got the best of me. I tried to do too much stuff all at once.

I don't think what I did is uncommon. I've seen it with a good friend who's going through cancer right now. My friend is doing the exact same thing: trying to work out too hard, thinking it's going to make a big difference. Overtraining taxes the immune system, decreasing the body's ability to recover during treatment.

This is where I stand on exercise and cancer: it's important that you save your energy. Move a little bit without pushing your immune system too far. Pay close attention to your white blood cell count when you get bloodwork done every two weeks or so.

Whenever possible use the stairs, if you can. But at some point, your heart's going to race, you're going to be out of breath, and you are going to feel too fatigued. I distinctly remember at some of the worst times I could barely keep my eyes just from the effects of the chemotherapy. I felt like a zombie from *The Walking Dead*.

At some point you're going find that you just don't have the energy or stamina when the chemotherapy kicks in. Then, one of the most powerful thing you can do, other than maintaining simple, disciplined movements, is to sleep. Take lots of naps. That's what your body is going to need to recover, especially if you're going through chemotherapy or anything toxic.

The next thing that's super important is that you drink water constantly. Lots of it.

Toxin-Removing Treatments

When facing cancer and undergoing chemotherapy, one of the things to do whenever possible is a holistic treatment or workout that will push your liver and squeeze toxins out of your body. For example, yoga.

Another treatment valuable treatment is the sauna, especially an infrared sauna. These have been proven beneficial to anyone who's going through cancer treatment.

Next are regular massages. That's a great way to get your lymph moving and try to instigate some white blood cell movement in your body. Also, acupuncture is a powerful way to help detoxify and improve circulation and energy flow inside the body.

Another potentially beneficial treatment, but you need to be cautious of this and certainly talk to your doctors about it, are enemas. I didn't do them because I had colorectal cancer. The biggest challenge with treatments involving the bowels is they can be extremely fatiguing. The amount of energy your digestive and elimination systems use is very high. And when you're getting lots of treatments, are on medications, and your body isn't absorbing nutrition effectively due to all the antibiotics, enemas or colonics can make this even worse.

My Morning Workout

Now that I've been clean and cancer-free for a couple years, I've made significant changes in my diet, my sleep, and my exercise and workout routines. I do a really good workout in 10 to 20 minutes a day. My body fat is down to approximately 11%. I am leaner and more muscular now than I was 15 years ago. In fact, I look younger today than I did 15 years ago because I got rid of the poisons, toxins, and inflammation in my body.

Before I share my workout routine, let me say that if you're undergoing treatment, it's probably not the right time to do this entire workout. Only do as much as you're comfortable doing.

The whole routine will take about 20 minutes. It's made me a happier person, a better person, and much more efficient.

Morning Gratitude

I begin with a morning gratitude ritual. I record in my journal five different ways I feel gratitude that morning. The next component is the positive inspirational saying that I repeat over and over that follows the phrase: "Today I am ... " For example, I could say, "Today I am ... an inspirational leader for my tribe." I repeat this several times. The system I use is called The Five Minute Journal—check it out in the Resources section of this book.

Deep Breathing

After I've got my mind moving, I take deep breaths. At this point, I try to do 50 deep breaths. To see how to do this breathing, look up online "Tony Robbins Priming," "Wim Hof breathing," "pranic breathing," or "Pranayama." It is diaphragmatic breathing through the nose. You inhale and exhale quickly to flood your body and brain with lots of oxygen. This has been scientifically proven to make you feel better and happier.

Deep Stretching

Next I stretch by bending forward, bringing my hand towards my toes, relaxing, and deeply breathing. Essentially, it's a deep hamstring stretch. I do it for approximately a minute or two. Each time I exhale, I bend over a little bit further until I can touch my toes. Stretching detoxifies the body.

Movement

Squats: I do 10 deep squats with my toes pointed forward, not "duck feet." Deep squats are good for the abdomen, for releasing gas, and and for flexibility. When you squat, you're engaging the biggest muscles in your body.

After completing each movement, I repeat the five things I am grateful for. So, that happens here and after every movement for a total of 5 repetitions of the 5 things I am grateful for.

Pushups: I do as many pushups as I can—around 50. When you start, you may only be able to do 5 deep squats and 5 pushups, and that's okay. Eventually you're going to increase these, so you can do 100 or more. Remember, as you do each pushup, you should breathe through your nose and activate your glutes and stomach muscles to strengthen your core.

Burpees: I do as many burpees as possible. Try to do at least 5. I have friends who can do 100 burpees at a time. This is a combination of squats, jumping, and pushups, and is one of the best strength-training exercises you can do without equipment.

Sprints: I'm fortunate that I live across the street from the ocean. I run along the beach every morning and do sprints barefoot in the sand. I am now doing 5 or 6 100-yard sprints as fast as I possibly can. It's high-intensity training that doesn't take long, but when you combine it with the other exercises, it's perfect.

Crunches: I started by doing only 5 or 10 crunches. Now I'm up to 50–75. If you have back problems, it's because your stomach and core muscles are weak. Crunches are the cure for most back issues.

Cold Plunge

I complete my morning routine exercise by doing a cold plunge in the ocean. I swim out in the waves, I submerge myself fully, and then I swim back. Even in the winter time. If you can't do this, try taking a cold shower, which is definitely going to wake you up. (Of course, I don't recommend doing anything in the cold when you are going through chemotherapy treatment and have cold sensitivity.)

I didn't start doing this intense workout until after I recovered physically. In the meantime, doing some basic stretching, breathing, some squats, and maybe some pushups or crunches will help get your body moving and move the lymph, which is good for your white blood cells and immune system. When you create movement, you release toxins.

From this morning routine, I've noticed a massive shift in my mental acuity, my attitude, and my overall wellbeing and happiness. It's even cured a spell of depression I found myself in after turning 50. I noticed I felt sad, and it's helped a ton.

I'm currently at approximately 120 days into doing this workout almost every single day, and my entire body has been completely transformed. In addition to my 11% body fat, my bone density is 55% higher than the average man my age, and best of all, my wife thinks I'm hot.

The other great thing about this workout is it doesn't require any equipment, gym, or membership. You can do it in a tiny space anytime and anywhere. In fact, I think I'm going to take a break right now from writing this book, and do 15 burpees.

Up next: I'm going to talk about some unexpected discoveries I made in terms of faith and the spirit.

Stepping into the Spiritual

The spiritual path is simply the journey of living our lives. Everyone is on a spiritual path; most people just don't know it.

—Marianne Williamson

I was raised a Catholic. I was sent to a Catholic school for 12 years, but I never remember resonating with Catholicism or the notion of organized religion. Ever. In fact, I would have considered myself an angry atheist for a long time, an agnostic for a lot longer, and an agnostic agnostic along the way. I certainly wasn't the kind of person who became a wishful Christian and asked God for special favors while I was going through my treatments. I was mad at religion and anything having to do with it.

However, experiencing cancer opened my eyes to the whole idea of deep compassion, empathy, and understanding.

I can remember when I was getting treated at Duke University, I stayed at a special home called Caring Bridge. It is much like a Ronald McDonald house except for adults. In that home, I was with other adults who were undergoing cancer treatment. Some of those people lived and others died.

Also I frequently came into contact with children who were going through cancer treatment. It broke my heart because they were enduring an emotional pain and a physical pain that I didn't feel any of them deserved or should ever have to endure. It greatly saddened me.

I can remember feeling empathy well inside me, and that transformed my life. For the first time I understood the concept of Christ consciousnesses and Jesus Christ through a completely different filter than I had previously experienced.

Now I wouldn't go so far as to call myself a Christian, but much like C.S. Lewis, I would consider myself an apologetic Christian. In other words, I feel connected to the principles and teachings. I also married a Jew, and I feel connected to Judaism as a culture.

The reason I'm telling you this is to point out that going through the cancer experience can awaken a part of you and open up your heart in ways that you may not have imagined before. You'll get the chance to connect with God and experience gratitude on a whole new level. It will allow you to appreciate every moment you have alive or that's remaining.

The great lesson here is that when you are in a state of gratitude, fear can't live inside you.

HeartMath

HeartMath is an institute that does research on the connection between the heart and the brain. From that, they've developed tools to help you harness this connection so that you can reduce your levels of stress and live healthier and happier.

Let me tell you about a HeartMath tool called Inner Balance that I swear by. It clips onto your ear and communicates to your phone using Bluetooth. From there, it allows you to learn how to regulate something called heart-mind coherence—the frequency of gratitude. It's a very simple process where you just look at the screen of your phone, you breathe in and out, all the while trying to synchronize your breathing with a deep sense of gratitude. The sensor measures your response and gamifies the experience to put you in a high state of gratitude. It's easy to do, and it has been proven to be extremely healthy to your brain and your body.

At HeartMath and other research centers scientists have proven that when you are in a state of gratitude or in heart-mind coherence, your body will heal faster. You will be more calm and more loving. Your IQ will actually improve. Plus, your stress levels will decrease by a measurable amount. Check the resources section for links.

The Five Minute Journal

Another tool that I highly recommend is The Five Minute Journal, available at Amazon and other places. (In the previous chapter I mentioned that it's what I use at the start of my morning gratitude ritual.)

The premise of The Five Minute Journal is to take five minutes in the morning and five minutes at night to explore gratitude through the question system the journal offers. Though it is brief, over time its effect is noticeable. It definitely increases your spiritual consciousness and improves the quality of your life.

Hoffman Process Revisited

I've already talked about the benefits of the Hoffman Process offered at the Hoffman Institute. Out of all the personal development work I've ever done, this week-long experience was the most valuable. Best of all, there are no gurus and no giant upsells. There's not a bunch of marketing going on. Instead, it plainly focuses on helping you increase and improve your spiritual consciousness.

The Power of the Collective

Finally, I highly recommend that you or your spouse join some kind of a group process or survivor group. It has been proven, especially with breast cancer, that people who get together and talk about their experiences live longer and are healthier.

When you're able to share your experiences and communicate your emotions, you're going to be a healthier person who lives longer and has a stronger sense of hope. At the end of the day, I believe spirituality is the process of experiencing hope and certainty. Giving yourself a sense of clarity, hope, and certainty will help you survive. I know, speaking for myself, it did for me.

Up next: the lowdown on surgery, chemotherapy, and radiation. I don't sugarcoat it, but I also relate the strategies I used to get me through it with the greatest ease possible.

Choosing Your Treatments

Hope is important because it can make the present moment less difficult to bear. If we believe that tomorrow will be better, we can bear a hardship today.

—Thich Nhat Hanh

My oncologist, Dr. Banerjee, told me that he'd own me for a year, and he was right.

When I was first diagnosed, I went through all the treatments: surgery, installation of a port, chemotherapy, and radiation. I can tell you that it really sucked, it really hurt, but there were a few things that got me through. Before I go into the treatments, let me tell you about those powerful coping mechanisms.

Mind Games

There were three mind games that I practiced on a regular basis that made a big difference.

The first: whether I was recovering from surgery or enduring chemotherapy or radiation, I'd say to myself, "If I can just get through this next minute … If I can just get through the next 5 minutes … If I can get through the next 10 minutes." In this way I divided the pain, and really the whole process, into more endurable moments that I could accomplish, that I could rack up under my belt as wins.

Another mindset I purposely took on was the vacationer's point of view. In my mind I'd act as if the entire cancer experience was a sort of vacation. I'd ask myself, "When's the last time I got to have 6 months or a year off? When have I ever had the luxury of taking so many naps, relaxing, and watching as many movies as I wanted to?" Sure, it wasn't all happy-go-lucky, but that's not the point. The point is creating an attitude of gratitude and seeing how even though the glass has cancer, it's still half full.

The third strategy that I've mentioned repeatedly already, but I have to revisit it because it's just so effective is the me-as-actor-in-movie game. I'd essentially move myself outside of my body, so I became an observer of the actor playing a person called "Mike." I would watch this Mike character as if through a camera, like his (my) life was a movie. Sure, a lot of the time the "movie" was just Mike (me) lying in the fetal position in bed, trying to stay comfortable and avoid any moving that would cause pain—not the most entertaining of films! But still, by getting outside myself and giving myself a little distance, even though it was just a mental thing, I found some freedom.

As long as I played these mind games, time went by surprisingly quickly. I even started to live outside of time. In other words, I started experiencing a lot of joy, just resting, relaxing, and floating in a cloud.

Treatments

I'm going to repeat what I told you at the very start of this book because it's just that important: the process of going through all of these treatments requires following a precise set of steps that your doctors will lay out for you. Follow your doctor's plan exactly and precisely.

As we already know, there's a possibility that the long-term damage and side effects from chemotherapy and radiation will cause cancer again in a person later on. Though there's this possibility, for me, I saw it as playing a statistics game and trying to increase my probability of survival.

As I already shared, I focused on short-term survival for the sake of my son, even if there could be long-term permanent damage from the short-term "fixes" I chose. I wanted to try any treatment my doctor recommended if it could increase my odds of survival in the short-term, even a little bit.

As I see it, medical science and genetic science are making discoveries and innovations so quickly that as long as you can live a little bit longer, there's a chance that some of the damage that's done to your body from a treatment can be reversed with new technology that's coming out. My advice is focus on your survival first and remember to go thermonuclear as quickly as possible.

On Surgery

This is how I describe the typical surgery experience. You go for surgery. Next you wake up, but you're still highly drugged, so you most likely waver in and out of pain for a while. That's what it is, and it takes you a certain period of time to recover, so your body starts functioning again.

In the case of recovering from colorectal cancer surgery, it took almost a week before I had my first poop. I was so excited to find out that I actually could poop again, but it hurt a lot. It took a while until my body started to function again properly.

Chemotherapy

After I healed from surgery, it was time for chemotherapy. The first thing was getting a port put in. (To this day I have a port scar.) Because chemotherapy administered via injections can destroy your veins, you get a port installed. Then they just stick a needle through that port, and you're hooked up.

For chemotherapy, they drain a variety of toxins inside you to kill the cancer. Of course, it also harms your immune system as well, and there's all the side effects. The aim is for the toxins to kill the cancer before the toxins (or the cancer) kill you.

Let's talk about those side effects. Hair loss: I remember waking up every day with a little bit of hair in my pillowcase. Very unpleasant. I know it can be even more unpleasant for a woman. Another side effect: you feel old, very weak, and exhausted. There can be nausea. A variety of pains. It's very common to have a lot of stomach problems and find it difficult to hold down food. You also start losing a sense of taste. You might have burning sensations inside your body, strange rashes, and all sorts of other unpleasantries.

Something to note is that there's often some kind of delay, for me it was a 3- or 4-day delay, after your chemotherapy treatment before you feel absolutely miserable. The reason why you don't feel miserable right away is because they oftentimes add steroids to your cocktail, which gives you a temporary boost. They may also do something to boost your white blood cells for a period of time. What does happen is eventually you experience a lot of energy loss. You may have insomnia or other side effects.

Here's what's important about chemotherapy: remind yourself that it's going to pass and that you're going to go through different cycles.

It can be helpful to keep a daily record of how you feel. You could have a chart on a scale of 1 to 10, for example. Then, when you are feeling absolutely miserable, you can look back to previous journal entries, where you tracked your daily progress after treatments, to remind yourself that yes, you eventually bounced back after feeling so awful before, so you'll do it again this time too.

Right about the time when you start feeling almost normal again is when you're going to go back for your next treatment. That's usually how it works.

In my case, I got a treatment every 2 weeks. Some people have to do it every day. Other people might go every 3 or sometimes every 4 weeks. If you're fortunate, you may just have oral chemotherapy, which will have a different set of side effects. Whatever the case, it's going to be unpleasant and it will eventually end.

If your chemotherapy results in you experiencing neuropathy, which is the lack of sensitivity to your fingers and toes, know that the neuropathy can be repaired later on with alpha-lipoic intravenous treatments. Definitely investigate those.

Radiation

Finally, radiation. I decided to do radiation treatment because it gave me an extra 7% chance of survival.

The place on your body you get the radiation will determine some of your side effects. My radiation was down in my groin area, so I experienced side effects down there. There was a fair amount of burning there, and it was not pleasant to pee or poop.

Given the fact that I already had terrible pain in my abdomen from the surgery and from colorectal cancer, the combination of all these treatments translated into me spending a lot of time visiting the toilet; on my worst day, 37 times. It got so bad that when I'd wipe my rear end, it was bleeding just from wiping.

As far as long-term side effects from radiation go, to this day I still haven't been tested to see if I'm still fertile or not, but most likely radiation down in my groin area made me completely infertile or not very fertile.

My summary on treatments: as long as you enter into your treatments every day with a smile on your face, gratitude that you're alive, and knowhow that you're going to get past this and it's going to get better, you'll make it. All you have to do is just get through the next 5 minutes. Play those mind games, and you'll be fine.

Up next: just like those mind games help you to manage the treatments with more ease, you'll also be prescribed painkillers. We'll explore the delicate balance of taking opiates.

Painkillers: A Delicate Balance

The greatest evil is physical pain.

—Saint Augustine

This chapter is all about drugs: pain-relieving opiates. Let me start by painting a picture of my life during this time.

A Day in the Life

I'd had the surgery already, and I was living in North Carolina at Duke University Clinic getting daily doses of oral chemotherapy and radiation.

I'd get up in the morning and shower. As I cleaned my body, I'd watch more hair go down the drain. When I went to make my bed, I started by picking the hair off my pillow, hair that had fallen out overnight. At this point, a lot of it had fallen out. My hair had turned almost completely gray. I was extremely thin and gaunt. After that, I'd put on my clothes and go to treatment.

For radiation I'd wear nothing more than a hospital gown and my cowboy boots. I've been wearing "Blunnies," Australian cowboy boots, for about 25 years, and even though I was supposed to wear hospital booties, the nurses let me wear my cowboy boots.

At this point the nurses who ran the radiation room thought I was a real character. I had a brand-new butt, poop, and fart joke for them every single day. They were heavy Southern women who loved to laugh, and I always did my very best to make them giggle and laugh as much as possible. Of course, I'd flash my butt and purposely not wear the backside of the hospital gown. Maybe some consider that sexual harassment, but it was funny as hell, especially in the South.

I'd lay down on the radiation platform and stuff my junk in a lead pan, so it wouldn't get damaged anymore than it already was. The nurses would put a little flag right around my but. Then they'd line up lasers with some permanent marker drawings that had been written all over my body to align the radiation treatment (to protect my private parts and my butthole from getting permanently damaged). The system would turn on, making some wild noise. From behind the leaded glass and shielding, the machine would give me life-saving, or life-threatening, depending on how you looked at it, radiation.

After a few minutes of being radiated, I would stand up, dress myself, and go see my doctor for a quick checkup. After that, I'd drive to a Whole Foods, where I would pick out a meal for the day. At that point I would be feeling okay because the fatigue hadn't gotten to me yet, and I hadn't taken my daily dose of oral chemotherapy. Because I didn't have anything in my stomach, I would have control over my bodily functions. But I knew what would be happening next.

I would return to the "adult Ronald McDonald House" where I was staying. I'd walk upstairs, take my oral chemo, and eat something. Generally speaking, within about 10 or 15 seconds, I'd have to make a run to the bathroom.

What was strange is the moment something hit my stomach, something else would have to come out. That would continue, between a few bites of food and more diarrhea, for a couple of hours.

Next, I would take a small dose of hydromorphone and a little bit of Lorazepam, also known as Ativan. The painkillers "took the edge" off the extreme fatigue and pain. Then I'd lie down, turn on my iPad, launch Netflix, and start watching movies with bathroom breaks every 5–10 minutes.

As time went on, there was more time between the bathroom visits. It got to be where they happened every 30 to 40 minutes.

A little bit later on, I'd eat a little bit more food, go through that same cycle, take another round of painkillers, and watch movies until I finally fell asleep, only to repeat the same pattern the next day.

While this was my life for about 2 months, as in I was taking multiple doses of painkillers every day for a couple months, it wasn't easy or natural for me to get into the practice. Really, it was the opposite.

My Drug History

Before Cancer

I grew up in an environment where drugs were bad, but alcohol was okay. As already shared, I drank pretty frequently starting from age 18 because it was legal. Not excessively, but regularly.

Growing up, my one and only drug experience was smoking marijuana at age 18. Just that one time. The result: a horrible reaction. I was hospitalized for about a week and a half with severe anxiety and paranoia attacks that continued for a year. For the next 3.5 years I had frequent flashbacks. Since then, I learned that I have a certain genetic predisposition that makes me susceptible to severe anxiety and paranoia if I have any CBD or marijuana inside my body. My brain doesn't like it.

Aside from that, I had never used any other drug my entire life—until cancer treatment. That's when, of course, they give you opiates.

During Cancer

Frankly, I was horrified that I would become an addict once they started giving me opiates in the hospital, so when I first had my treatments, surgery and chemotherapy, I avoided taking painkillers. I was very afraid I would become addicted, and I didn't want that to happen, so I muscled my way through the pain.

Looking back, I'm not sure that this was a good thing or a bad thing, but I can tell you that one of the biggest benefits that painkillers will give you is a chance for your brain and your body to do what they need to do. Your body needs to heal, and your brain needs to be separated from the pain, so your body can heal. In other words, when you are using painkillers responsibly, your won't experience and feel the pain, so your body can do what it needs to do, which is to heal.

I believe I actually *caused* trauma to my brain and I healed more slowly by *not* taking the drugs. Once I realized this I starting taking the opiates I'd been prescribed.

The Delicate Balance

The problem, of course, is managing the delicate balance between responsibly taking the painkillers and getting addicted. Based on the rapid opioid crisis we're seeing worldwide, it doesn't appear as though most people manage that balance very well.

Opiates are habit-forming, and most people like them. Of course, there are people who don't like them because they can make you feel itchy and a bit weird. Plus, they can make you constipated.

When I have very honest conversations with survivors after they've had cancer treatments and taken opiates, they admit that they miss the them. Also some admit that they continue to take them on a frequent basis. That's an unfortunate reality in our world today. It's pretty easy to buy them when you're outside of the country. For example, you can to go Mexico and buy opiates easily at a pharmacy if you ask for them.

Whatever the case, I think it's important that you're honest with yourself because denial and being dishonest with yourself and your doctors are what get you into trouble. So if you like them, tell yourself the truth, that you like them. Just don't overdo them.

You will have cravings, after the fact. It's normal. You simply must find a way to manage your cravings. Make sure you tell your doctors the truth. They know how to deal with this. Talk to your therapist about them as well. For example, your doctor can supply you with a less addictive and weaker drug, like codeine, if you do have real pain.

Never mix alcohol with painkillers because a cocktail can cause respiratory failure.

There is a non-addictive painkiller that I've found effective. It is called kratom, and a brand name I've used is Krabot. It is a natural herb. There are some people trying to legislate against it, but it is currently legal. You can buy it online.

I still have an extremely sensitive stomach and system. Occasionally if I have a severe diarrhea attack when I eat something my body doesn't agree with, I will be hobbled for hours with intestinal challenges. Kratom has given me a non-addictive option that I've found to be effective at dealing with the pain.

Up next: I chose to go thermonuclear against the cancer, cutting, blasting, and burning it out of me. Even still, there's a place for alternative and integrative therapies as well.

Recovery: Integrative and Alternative Treatments

Medicine is a science of uncertainty and an art of probability.

—William Osler

When I got my diagnosis, my aim was short-term survival. So, I put my faith in allopathic medicine first, meaning going in and blasting and killing that cancer.

I didn't want to take on an integrative regimen at the same time because I worried it would interfere with the treatments my oncologist had recommended. I wasn't going to risk following any potentially airy fairy treatments that could put my life at risk.

Multiple oncologists advised me not to take any nutritional supplements or do anything outside their allopathic regimens because it could interfere with the chemotherapy. For example, if I were to do an alternative therapy that aimed to strengthen a part of my system that the oncologists were trying to essentially weaken in order to kill the cancer, then it could be counterproductive. Disastrous even. This made a lot of sense.

After Detonating the H-Bomb

First let me repeat: I'm not a doctor. I don't play one on the Internet or on TV, so consult your medical doctor before doing any alternative treatment. If there's a tiebreaker to be made, don't listen to me.

With that said, it's my opinion that you should first go thermonuclear on your cancer, depending on what stage it is, of course. Once you've done that, then use alternative and integrative therapies that work in concert with your allopathic regimen. I'm not an advocate for one or the other. I'm an advocate for both. But I think there is appropriate timing for both.

What I wish for myself is that I'd incorporated alternative and integrative therapies sooner. As it stands, I have a certain degree of neuropathy and damage that's occurred to my body that I still haven't fully counteracted. To this day, I live with numbness in my fingers and toes. I still have an extremely sensitive stomach.

Just how sensitive is my stomach? If I go to a restaurant and eat some salad or some kind of food (you see, I still haven't figured all this out), within a couple of minutes I have to make a dash for the toilet. In fact, sometimes I can take a bite of food and immediately my stomach starts to gurgle; that's when I know I'm in trouble. It's that fast. From there, I might have 5 to 7 minutes before I'm going to the toilet.

Frankly, it's very unsettling and embarrassing to be at a restaurant with friends, and over the course of the meal, I've got to go to the bathroom 4 or 5 times. I will literally be completely eliminated by the time I walk out of there. Not only that, I'm miserable, I'm so tired and beat because my bowels have sapped all my energy. Those are the instances where I may end up having to take some kind of a painkiller just to alleviate the challenges.

These "residual effects" are what make me wish I'd incorporated alternative and integrative therapies into my recovery much sooner than I did. Perhaps I could've prevented or else lessened it by a lot. So, now, what I recommend is the following.

I recommend finding an integrative medical professional who can work with you and with your allopathic team of doctors.

My integrative medical professional is the amazing Dr. Nalini Chilkov. Several people I know and esteem recommended her. When I finally met her, she shook my hand and told me, "I know who you are. I followed your work for years."

Surprised and feeling a bit exposed, I ventured to ask, "Are you're going to have to look at me naked?"

She shook her head, assuring me, "No, I'm not that kind of doctor."

Nalini was a godsend. Her specialty is working with patients who have cancer. She consults closely with their oncologists, surgeons, chemotherapy doctors, and/or radiation oncologists to ensure her recommended therapies don't compromise any allopathic treatments and can actually work in tandem with them.

Other alternative treatments I recommend include herbal or Chinese therapies, acupuncture, and massage. Of course you must talk with your oncologist about alternative treatments you're interested in to make sure you'll be helping yourself and not interfering with the allopathic treatments.

Testing

You can't treat or prevent a disease if you don't diagnose it properly. In any area of science, technology, or medicine, you need testing and diagnosis.

This is a snapshot of a "blood work" order I'm getting 5 years after my initial diagnosis. I'm showing this to illustrate what extensive versus simple blood tests look like. When you see an oncologist, they only check a few points of data. When you do extensive blood work, you see a lot more, so you learn a lot more.

Why do so many oncologists say something ignorant like "It doesn't matter what you eat while you're getting chemo"? It's because they're looking at a few data points instead of dozens. Your blood doesn't lie.

Description	CPT	ICD10	Description	CPT	ICD10
CMP 14	80050		Fibrinogen activity	85384	D68.69
CBC + DIFF +PLAT	85025		D-Dimer	85378 85379	D68.69
UA Complete	81005,81015		Galectin-3	82777	
hs CRP	86141	R79.82	LDH Lactic Acid Dehydrogeniase	82607	T45.1
NMR Profile+Insulin Resistance Markers	80061 83704	E78.5 E88.81	GGPT Gamma Glutamyl Transferase	82977	R94.5
Advanced Lipid Panel	80061, 83704, 82172, 83695, 83721	E78.5	MTHFR DNA Analysis	2770831	E72.11 E72.12
Omega 3.6 Fatty Acids	82542	E78.5	1140916 IL-6 Interleukin-6 plasma	83520	R53.8
Homocysteiene	83090	E72.11	905036 Transforming Growth Factor Beta-1	83520	
HgbA1c	83036	E88.81	Thyroid Panel hsTSH T4 T3 FTI	84443,84480 84436,84439, 84481	E06.3
Fasting Insulin	83525, 83527	E88.81	Free T3	601141 84481	E06.3
IGF-1 Insulin Like Growth Factor-1	84305		Free T4	601142 84439	E06.3
RBC Magnesium	683748	E83.42	Reverse T3	84482	E06.3
Vitamin D 25-OH	82306	E55.9	Serum Selenium	84255	E59
Vitamin D 1, 25 OH	82652	E55.9	002139 CEA	82378	R97.0
Vitamin B12	82607	D51.9	002261 CA 19-9	86301	R97.8
Folate	82746	E53.8	143404 CA 15-3	86300	R97.8
Iron, IBC	83550	E61.1	140293 CA 27.29	86300	R97.8
Ferritin	82728	E61.1	002303 CA-125	86304	R97.1
Serum Copper	82525	E83.0	PSA Total + Free	84154,84153	N41.0
Ceruloplasmin	82390	E83.0	Total+Free Testosterone	84403 84402	N95.1
Serum Zinc	84630	E60	DHEA-Sulfate	82627	N95.1
Urine Cross Linked N Telopeptide	82523 82570	M85.8	Estradiol	82670	N95.1
Progesterone	84133	N95.1	Estrone Sulfate	82679	N95.1
Pregnenolone	84140	N95.1	SHBG Sex Hormone Bindnig Globulin	84270	N95.1
117021 VEGF Serum	83520		Vitamin B6	84207	E53.1
Methylmalonic Acid	83921	E53.8	Thyroid Auto Antibodies anti TG, antiTPO	86376 86800	E06.9
DiHydroTestosterone	80327	N40.1	104018 Cortisol AM	82533	R53.8

When you work with your doctors, ask them if they'll do extensive blood testing and also find a good integrative or functional medical doctor that can look through the reports for additional details about your condition. The more data you have to work with, the more options you have for greater health.

Genetic Profile

Whether you have cancer or not, I highly recommend you get a genetic profile. There are many companies offering personal genetic testing nowadays, including Color Genomics, Ancestry.com, 23andMe, and Promethease. Each offers differing depths of results, so you should investigate to see which you prefer.

Another resource is scientist Dr. Rhonda Patrick from www.FoundMyFitness.com, who has appeared on *The Tim Ferriss Show* and several other podcasts, also offers personal genetic testing to uncover advanced data related to cancer, immunotherapy, and beyond. You can upload your results from your 23AndMe profile into her system and learn all sorts of interesting things about your body that you can't get from a normal or extensive blood test.

The reason I recommend getting a genetic test is because you can learn about your genetic disease predispositions (among other things). For example, as I already mentioned, I learned that I have a genetic predisposition that is 1.4 times higher than the average person for getting colorectal cancer. I also have an 8-time higher probability of getting type 1 diabetes than the average person, which is very high. There are other genetic predispositions I have that can cause me to have a higher probability of getting or different types of diseases or cancers as well.

Technology

I've recently invested in some technology that allows an Apple Watch to read and register my EKG information. Personally, I don't like wearing watches but because this device measures EKG, I'm going to regularly check my EKG and store my heart data and all of my health information, so it can be monitored. I believe predictive medicine is a massive opportunity for us to live longer, healthier, higher-quality lives.

So bottom line is this: connect with an integrative or functional medical doctor now before you're sick, assuming you aren't. If you're going through cancer, connect with an integrative doctor, get some referrals, and look inside my references for some possible treatments. My advice would be to get acupuncture, get massages, and get extensive tests, like the ones from LabCorp and others that I will provide information about in the Resources section.

Other Aspects of Recovery

A lot of the stuff here, I've mentioned already in other contexts in this book. Because these things are so valuable, let's revisit them in the context of recovering from cancer.

Because of the long-term traumatic side effects of the drugs and treatments, I highly recommend seeing a therapist to help you process everything as well as undergoing the Hoffman Process.

Investigate J. J. Virgin's books and the Virgin Diet. She is an honest-to-goodness nutritionist and one of my best friends. I trust her implicitly and explicitly.

If you are looking to take supplements, one of the best quality nutritional supplement companies is Designs for Health. I personally know the CEO and founder of that organization, Jonathan Lizotte. His products are of the highest quality.

The other thing to do is research additional ways to boost your immune system and your stomach biome via natural means. This will include using probiotics and other supplements.

Another possibility to investigate are after-the-fact stem cell treatments. In this area I'm working with a gentleman named Dr. Matthew Cook. His contact information is also available in the Resources section from this book as well.

At the very least, the big things that will make the most significant difference in your recovery include drinking lots of water and eating a high-quality diet like the one described earlier in the book.

Up next: the time will come when you get to return to work. Harness all the insights you've gained from this cancer ordeal and use that to shape a new worklife.

Returning to Work

A rebirth out of spiritual adversity causes us to become new creatures.

—James E. Faust

When you return to work, you'll find it very easy to fall back into your old routine and addiction of working too hard. You shouldn't need me to tell you that that will get you nowhere very quickly. The last thing you need is to get sick again, so don't overestimate your body, your brain, or the trauma that has been inflicted on it.

When I returned, I didn't have a lot of energy, and I was often on the toilet. I ended up needing to take lots of naps. If you are working at an office, just make sure you've got somewhere where you can lie on your back and take catnaps.

Continue relying on your team. Continue asking for help. Consider getting an outsource business manager or some low-cost labor to help take the load off of some administrative duties and tasks. The bottom line: make sure you continue to ask for help.

Little Hinges

What made a huge difference for me is I came back with a plan. I came back with goals. I created a goal sheet. I focused on moving big rocks to gain leverage. Remember the old saying: big doors swing on little hinges.

When I came back after cancer treatment, I realized that if I was going to continue running the business, it would kill me. I didn't want that to happen. So that's where my plan came in.

I brought in a very good friend who helped me package my business and prepare it for sale. We were fortunate enough to package the business in a way so that we could sell it to a publicly traded company. For me, it was the second time I exited.

Doing this required an enormous amount of preparation and work, but what we did is we focused on increasing the value of the business in how we packaged it. This wasn't easy to do because a lot of my products and services depended on my unique set of skills and talents. However, because the business had been flourishing while I was gone, I learned more about how to package and prepare it.

If you can package your information or business in such a way that it can be licensed, that's going to do a lot for you. It'll give you a chance to recover on your own terms instead of someone else's.

A New Filter

Let me explain to you a very important concept that made a massive difference to me psychologically. Several years ago my good friend Ed Rush challenged me to see my role through a new filter. Here's how he did it.

Ed told me the following: if you think about it, there are generally 2,000 working hours in a year. If you want to make $100,000 per year, that works out at $50 per hour for those 2,000 hours. Realistically, it's probably closer to 1,000 billable working hours a year, so that makes the rate $100 per hour.

What that means then is that any task that's around you that you can hire someone to do for $50 an hour or less, you want to outsource it. Or again, if you're realistic about the billable hours, anything that is $100 an hour or less, you want to outsource. Yes, I know that you have to take into consideration your cost of doing business, marketing costs, taxes, etc., but precision isn't what's important here. It's the big idea.

Let's upscale it and say your goal is to make $1,000,000 per year, that would translate into $500 or $1,000 per hour.

Ed's point to me, and my point to you, is this: be very selective about what you choose to actually do yourself. When you do the math, most tasks aren't worth your time or money—so don't do them. You need to outsource as much as possible, especially while you're sick. Remember too that when I was going through treatment and only had an hour per day of "useful" energy to work, my companies were actually MORE profitable than when I was in them!

After cancer, especially, you need to look at your business through a new filter. Very likely, some of the stuff that got you in trouble and made you sick in the first place was probably due to inflammation, which was probably caused by stress or the lifestyle you were living as an overworked entrepreneur.

When you do the math, you'll see that really you only need to do a select number of tasks. Most of the stuff you are chasing your tail to get done, it makes the most financial (and health and wellbeing) sense to outsource or delegate.

If you're going to prevent cancer and illness from ever happening to you again, it's very important that you learn how to change your lifestyle and change your thinking. Only then can you evolve into the next best version of you.

What will ultimately happen when you return back to work, if you can stay connected with your compassion, passion, and new zest for life that hopefully cancer has caused you to reconnect with, is you're going to find some positive ways to change your life around. You're going to find that you're a much more effective, efficient, loving, caring, and compassionate person. Use that to put the good kind of pressure on yourself that will help you return back to work in a healthy way where you've actually change your lifestyle too.

Up next: we're nearing the end ... well, sort of. Check out the resources and interviews that come up after the following Final Thoughts.

Final Thoughts

You may not realize it when it happens, but a kick in the teeth may be the best thing in the world for you.
—Walt Disney

Based on my personal experience and in speaking with a lot of other survivors and people going through it, cancer can actually be a significant gift, one that will change your life.

What I believe is most important is that you trust the process. You ask lots of great questions. You make a decision, you execute quickly, and you don't waiver. Don't second guess. Even if it doesn't feel good and you want to quit, finish the process.

Your doctors have lots of experience and will guide you down the right path, as long as you ask really good questions and tell them everything. Tell them what you're feeling. Tell them what you're thinking, what you're experiencing. Give them lots and lots of details.

Doctors will take a greater interest in you if you take a big interest in your treatments. When you read my interviews with survivors, you'll find they say the same thing.

Get an advocate to work alongside you. That can be a spouse, a parent, or a good friend who looks out for your best interest.

Food matters. Don't listen to people who aren't nutritionists. Those doctors don't know what they're talking about when it comes to food (unless they are looking at detailed blood reports that are far beyond what you're going to get from a normal oncologist).

Use integrative, naturopathic treatments, as long as they don't interfere with your standard allopathic treatments. In other words, allow your doctors to overrule your integrative medical professionals if they don't agree on something.

Next, consider some of the resources and tools that I recommend and that the survivors whom I interview recommend. Remember, I will be transparent. That means that in some cases, like Bulletproof, for example, I reveal that I have a financial interest in the company. I do not recommend anything that I don't personally use or believe in. That's because I invest in people and programs that work, and I spend a lot of time finding and searching for the best of the best of the best.

The only other thing that you'll want to do is head over to the membership site at www.Cancerpreneur.com and take advantage of the resources and tools offered. Feel free to share any of this information with someone in need of hope, courage, confidence, resources, and tools. Share it with anyone looking for a way to go through the cancer process and survive with their marriage, family, and business intact.

Please take a moment to review this book on Amazon, and give it your honest opinion. If there's something that you don't like, please share that by sending me a direct email. All my contact information is listed below.

Resources

American Institute of Integrative Oncology Research and Education: https://www.aiiore.com/
Dr. Nalini Chilkov's education and courses for healthcare professionals to become informed on how to support cancer patients' overall health—before, during, and after cancer.

Mike Anderson's *Healing Cancer from Inside Out*: http://amzn.to/2BS79K0
    *Recommended by Hal Elrod

Cancerpreneur: www.Cancerpreneur.com
Go here to find free resources, tools, interviews, and updates.

Caring Bridge: https://www.caringbridge.org/
This is a platform where you can post your cancer updates and progress, so that you can manage communications with your community in a simple, effective way.

Dr. Matthew Cook, MD, and head of BioReset Medical, Regenerative Medicine Specialist in Campbell, CA: www.BioResetMedical.com
This is the doctor I'm working with to restore my gut and eliminate neuropathy and other side effects using experimental stem cells.

Gratitude Process: https://thehustle.co/the-five-minute-journal-will-make-you-happier

Here is an article describing the efficacy of The Five Minute Journal.

HeartMath Inner Balance: https://store.heartmath.com
This is a device that can help you relax, meditate, and achieve "heart mind coherence."

The Hoffman Process:
https://www.hoffmaninstitute.org/
I believe this is the most powerful personal development resource for forgiveness, hope, and spiritual growth. It is NOT religious. There are no gurus, cults, upsells or crazy communities. Just good solid psychology.

Integrative Cancer Answers:
http://www.integrativecanceranswers.com/
"Integrative Cancer Answers is the fruit of Dr. Nalini Chilkov's 30 years of experience transforming the cancer journey for thousands of patients worldwide. Her OutSmart Cancer Plans are recognized as the most comprehensive, safe and effective doctor-designed programs available today."

Mike Koenig's Contact Info:
    Facebook Wall: https://www.facebook.com/Koenigs
    Email: MikeKoenigs@gmail.com

LabCorp: https://www.labcorp.com/
This is where I get extensive blood work done.

Dr. Rhonda Patrick, PhD:
https://www.foundmyfitness.com/
She offers personal genetic testing to uncover advanced data related to cancer, immunotherapy, and more.

Rev.com: https://www.rev.com/

> This is an app and service that you can use to make audio and video recordings, and then if you choose, you can also get them transcribed.

Tony Robbins Priming:
https://www.youtube.com/watch?v=hBP-YBX597s
> This a great way to learn how to do that deep diaphragmatic nose breathing that I describe in my morning fitness routine.

TapeACall: https://www.tapeacall.com/

> This app records your incoming and outgoing iPhone calls. You can even coordinate with Rev.com to get them transcribed, if you want.

Vivian's Just Like My Child Foundation:
https://www.justlikemychild.org/

Books

Note: the Amazon short links are affiliate links. I think Amazon will pay me about $0.02 if you buy something AND I donate all of the income to charity.

> Dr. Nalini Chilkov's *32 Ways to OutSmart Cancer: How to Create a Body Where Cancer Cannot Thrive*:
> http://amzn.to/2BnRHsR

The Five Minute Journal: http://amzn.to/2B82Ii1
> This is a great tool to keep your mind in a positive, grateful state.

Louise Hay's *You Can Heal Your Life*:
> http://amzn.to/2AIMpFd
> "The author has a great deal of experience and firsthand information to share about healing, including how she cured herself after being diagnosed with cancer."

Dr. Kelly A. Turner's *Radical Remission: Surviving Cancer Against All Odds*: http://amzn.to/2kHQVQm
> "Dr. Kelly A. Turner, founder of the Radical Remission Project, uncovers nine factors that can lead to a spontaneous remission from cancer—even after conventional medicine has failed."

Verne Varona's *Nature's Cancer Fighting Foods*:
> http://amzn.to/2nLOf5C
> "Based on a solid foundation of the healing properties of good nutrition, this book empowers readers with the information they need to make the best choices and to gain control over their total health and well-being."
> * Recommended by David Wagner

J. J. Virgin's *The Virgin Diet: Drop 7 Foods, Lose 7 Pounds, Just 7 Days*: http://amzn.to/2ACkXcd
J. J. Virgin's book about eliminating inflammatory foods.

Doctor Interview: Nalini Chilkov

Dr. Nalini Chilkov, LAc, OMD, is a leading-edge authority and pioneer in the field of integrative cancer care, cancer prevention, and immune enhancement.

She is the founder of the American Institute of Integrative Oncology (www.AIIOre.com), providing professional and practical clinical training to frontline clinicians and the site www.IntegrativeCancerAnswers.com, providing resources for patients and families. She is the author of the #1 bestselling book 32 Ways to OutSmart Cancer: How to Create a Body Where Cancer Cannot Thrive.

Dr. Chilkov brings over 30 years of clinical experience, combining the best of functional medicine and oriental medicine. She has lectured at the School of Medicine at UCLA and UC Irvine in California and the Medical Academy in London, UK. She featured as a cancer expert on TAPIntegrative.com and on NBCTV, and has been recognized as one of the Top 10 Online Influencers for Breast Cancer by Dr. Mehmet Oz and WebMD. Her private practice is in Santa Monica, California.

Mike Koenigs: I am here with Dr. Nalini Chilkov, a specialist in integrative oncology. I credit Dr. Chilkov for nursing me back to health, especially in terms of my recovering from surgery, chemotherapy, and radiation. I have my beautiful body to thank for that, but I really have you to thank for that, so thank you for being here, Dr. Chilkov.

Why don't you give everyone your background, what it is specifically that you do?

Dr. Chilkov: One of the questions people often ask is "How did you get into this?" I got interested early in my life because of my family risk factors. Both of my parents were diagnosed with cancer in their 50s. However, when they both eventually died—my mom died at 88, my dad at 90—they died cancer-free.

For the last 30 years, I've been specializing in putting together teams of cancer-care professionals—that might include a patient's oncologist, radiologist, or surgeon—because you need both a disease expert and a health expert when you have a complex illness; plus the fact that in oncology, in particular, there's no health plan. There's no health model.

What do you want as a patient? You want your life back. You want health as your endpoint, but if there's no plan for that, then that's not where you're going. That's the piece I bring to the table.

MK: One of the scariest things that happens when a person gets a cancer diagnosis—and it happened to me— is you get the diagnosis, and suddenly, out of the woodwork everyone comes out. You don't know what the heck to believe. You've got every pill pusher and MLM fraudster out there, claiming they've got some cure. Then you've got people who are totally anti-traditional medicine, and then people who are on the opposite end. Then you look things up on Google, not that Google can cure cancer. So how does a person make a decision?

What you do, and you did for me, is you bridged that gap. What you bring to the table is you were able to communicate with my oncologist, who thinks everything that isn't traditional science and medicine is worthless (even though he's a third-generation doctor from an Indian family and from an Ayurvedic background). He's like, "Anything that I can't measure on a blood test is poppycock."

Dr. C: I think we all have to remember that every person who's our care provider wants the same good outcome for us. We have to understand that's the good motivation of even the most close-minded doctor—they still want the best for us. We have to remember that's where they're coming from.

In my experience, a lot of oncologists will say, "That doesn't work" or "That doesn't make a difference" or "Your diet doesn't count," because they're actually thinking food doesn't cure cancer.

What we want to understand is where they're coming from and then educate them by saying, "No, of course. I'm not claiming that pomegranates cure cancer. What we're trying to do is add another layer of support."

The oncologist is fascinated with your tumor, with your cancer, so we want to pick that person's brain and get everything they know about what to do to reduce your tumor burden.

They are not interested in what we call the "cancer terrain" or the "tumor microenvironment." That's where diet, lifestyle, herbs, and supplements come in to synergize and improve your chances for a really good outcome and to deal with some of the toxic effects of your treatments so that you have a plan for recovery.

I think a lot of oncologists think that a patient like you might consult with someone like me to abandon chemotherapy, radiotherapy, or surgery, but actually what you're doing is putting together the piece that the oncologist doesn't do, which is to support your health.

There's two metaphors that I use. One is the "soil in the garden metaphor." That is, if you change the soil in the garden, you change what grows there. In the same way, if you change that terrain or environment of the cells in your body, you change the behavior of cancer cells. That's a piece of what we're doing.

There's also the complexity of that cancer physiology, that's what the second metaphor addresses. Imagine a wheel with many spokes on it, and every spoke on that wheel is part of this complexity. The oncologist knows every spoke on that wheel, but because of their toxic toolbox, they can only pick one or two of those spokes. If you want to have a truly comprehensive approach, then you have to address the whole wheel, so we can do that.

MK: In your 30+ years doing this work, how many patients do you think you've worked with and helped?

Dr. C: I've been in practice almost 35 years now, and I've worked with thousands of patients.

I have also made an effort to create collaborative relationships with oncologists, oncology groups, surgeons, and radiologists because that's how the patient gets the best care, if everyone on their team is talking with each other. I think that that's really important.

For example, you're an entrepreneur. You're a person with your own original mind and thinking and sense of agency. When you put a team together, I think it's really important to realize you're the head of the team. The oncologist is not the head of the team. You want to put together a team of clinicians who respect your values and wishes for yourself. If you have medical care providers that do not do that, that speak down to you, infantilize you, or are control freaks, then that's not the way to have a healthy relationship with anyone.

MK: Let's pretend you get a call from an entrepreneur and they're diagnosed with some form of cancer. They've been recommended a combination of surgery, chemo, and radiation. The person confesses, "I'm not comfortable with doing all these treatments, but I can do some of them. However, I don't know how to communicate with my family and with the doctors to negotiate." What do you say?

Dr. C: The very first thing I say is "Take a breath." No one's prepared for this. It's completely overwhelming. A cancer diagnosis, whether it's stage 1 or stage 4, is not an emergency.

It's not an urgent care diagnosis. Cancer is a chronic illness. In the same way that you might be diagnosed with high blood pressure or high cholesterol or diabetes, you must think of it as a long-term project that you're going to figure out how to manage properly.

It's not an emergency, even though the oncologist may have said to you, "We've diagnosed you. Next week, we're starting chemo. Then after that, we'll do surgery. Then we'll do more chemo. Then we'll do radiation. Then maybe we'll do hormonal therapy. We're starting next week." That's completely unfair to any adult, number one.

If you have anything complex happening in your health, you should have a second and, perhaps, a third opinion. You should go on a learning curve. It should be your decision, not your oncologist's decision. You absolutely have to feel comfortable with it. That is key to a good outcome.

You have to trust the person caring for you also.

It's always my wish that someone comes into an office like mine at that juncture. That's not always when someone comes in, but if you come in at that place, then you can take a breath.

Allow yourself some time for your psyche to catch up to what just was diagnosed. Get your children and family in order. Sit down, have a family meeting. Find out who your real support system is. Get your business handled. You do not have to start treatment next week. It won't make or break your outcome.

In a larger context, let's say you've started treatment and you're in the middle of chemo. You're on a schedule of chemo and you're just worn-out. You're not ready for the next chemo. You actually have the choice to say to the oncologist, "I need a break. I need an extra week."

A lot of patients feel that if they do that, they will have an unsuccessful treatment, but there's no magic schedule. There's no magic number of treatments.

The best care is individualized care. If you become a very educated patient and you have an advocate, then you can go to the oncologist as an educated patient and say, "I need a rest. I can't do this next week. I want to wait an extra week." It's important to feel like you can do that and to feel like you're not putting your life at risk by doing that. That's the psychology that happens.

It's very important to speak up and communicate with your care providers and let them know exactly what's happening to you so that the treatment schedule and the dosing can all be tailored to you.

MK: What can happen is a person can get one side saying one thing and the other side saying something else—again, the sides are integrative versus traditional, allopathic medicine—so you feel torn.

For me, in the end, I gave the allopathic docs a higher score, and I was afraid to do the integrative. The oncologists were telling me, "Don't take any vitamins. Don't take any supplements. Don't do anything else."

What do you say to people who are concerned or afraid of this tie-breaking situation?

Dr. C: Just like anything in life, going into black-and-white thinking is never a great thing to do. When you are diagnosed with an advanced cancer, as you were, fear drives a lot of your decisions. Fear is never a good place to make major decisions from. Again, taking a little more time is important.

I think 11 second opinions, like what you got, is too much because then you put yourself into overwhelm, but that's you. My job is to help people make decisions. If you had come to me at the beginning, I would've encouraged you to have the conventional treatment and I would've supported you through that. That's what would've happened.

I would not have told you not to have the treatment that you had because, in your case, conventional oncology treats your type of cancer well. I get patients who come to me who actually don't want to do conventional oncology and much of the time, I say, "It should be part of your plan."

Here's how to think about it. Black-and-white thinking is not useful ever, and a lot of oncologists are in black-and-white thinking, as yours was. "Don't do anything else. I want to control everything that happens." Now, that's out of your doctor's good motivation to not want anything messed up when he knew he had a good solution for you.

My job, when a person is going through chemotherapy, radiotherapy, and surgery, is to help you to stay healthy during that stressful time, to mitigate the toxic and adverse effects of your treatment, allowing you to get the therapeutic benefit of the treatment, but also protecting your. Let's protect your nerves. Let's protect your kidneys. Let's protect your liver. Let's protect your brain. Let's protect your digestive tract. Let's make sure that your nutritional status is optimized.

Most chemotherapy goes in cycles. Chemotherapy is active for about 4 or 5 days, and then you have a break until your next chemo. In that break time, a lot can be done with nutrition, herbs, and vitamins. During those 4 or 5 days when the chemo is active, I withhold the nutrients that would interact. You want to have someone like me who's an expert with drug-nutrient, drug-herb interactions, but you also want to be supported.

Let me tell you a story about an advanced cancer patient I recently had. She's an ovarian cancer patient who had metastasis to her lungs and her brain, stage 4. She came in having lost about a third of her muscle mass and body weight. As a result, she was extremely weak. She wasn't actually going to be able to finish her treatment, and she's young. She's only in her 40s. That was extreme. She was not doing well, failure to thrive.

I put her on a very aggressive nutritional protocol. Not a cancer treatment protocol, but a nutritional protocol. In 2 weeks, she gained back 15 pounds of muscle because we turned off the part of her physiology that was digesting her muscle mass. Her oncologist was stunned.

That allowed her to be a healthier, more robust patient who could finish her treatment, which she did. She had an extraordinary response to her treatment, so her oncologist feels that she's an outlier. She did better than other patients.

My wish for my patients is they be the outliers. How are you going to defy the odds? How are you going to do better than the average patient?

Oncology is just targeting your tumor cells. It's a very stressful, energy-demanding, high-nutrient-demanding journey, as you well know. If you have support doing that, you could actually live a fairly normal life, feel well, but remember, the most important thing is your nutritional status. You need to protect your digestive function. If you have no appetite, if you feel nauseous, if you're having diarrhea, you don't even feel like eating, then you need to get that handled. My job during that part is to support and protect healthy, normal functioning so that you do well. That's an example.

MK: In your 35 years of practice, you've seen a lot of people who've survived and those who haven't. In your experience, what are the common traits of people who blast through cancer versus those who don't survive?

Dr. C: One of my colleagues wrote a book called *Radical Remission*, where she did hard research on that. She uncovered

9 factors. I don't remember them all, but I'll tell you from my own experience directly.

Number one, patients who are all-in, like you, are the outliers. If someone is halfway committed to their own wellbeing and health, then they have halfway results, so you have to be all-in. I ask my patients to do really hard things, as you know. You just have to drop your resistance and be all-in because you're saving your own life. Oncology is not magic. You have to have all the conditions that cause health, so that's really what you're asking me. Being all-in, doing things that are life-giving, and really looking at your habits, your self-sabotage, and the things that cause you to make unhealthy choices because this is about the rest of your life. This isn't just about right now when you're going through chemo.

Really having a love of life, having a good support system, and being willing to change—change your habits, change your diet, and take herbs and supplements. Studies show that patients that do that have better outcomes.

You have an extraordinarily high need for rest and getting enough exercise. Studies show that patients who exercise have better outcomes than patients who don't.

One of my colleagues, Dr. Keith Block, an integrative oncologist in Chicago, puts his patients on a treadmill while they're getting their IV chemo infusion as a way to show you're not convalescent just because you're being treated for cancer.

You should maintain a healthy lifestyle and fitness level, and attend to the things that have meaning for you. Studies actually show if you're really clear on your core values and what has meaning, then you are more likely to make choices congruent with that.

Many people say, "Cancer is the best thing that ever happened to me," which seems very paradoxical, but if you engage in the process as this gateway in your life with the potential for growth, insight, and transformation, and you take the opportunity to really look at what your priorities are, those people make big life changes as a result of going through this. They really change their lives, get out of unhealthy relationships, change their work, change their lifestyles, stop eating junk food, and really get in alignment with themselves.

It's about the capacity to be radically honest with yourself and to do hard things. Change and healing are synonymous. Transformation and healing are synonymous. This is an extraordinary opportunity to heal, not just to deal with cancer, but to heal your life. How we live has more impact on our health than anything in a bottle.

MK: Let's say it's an entrepreneur undergoing treatment, and they've got to manage the family, the spouse, and the business. What are your recommendations when the business revolves around them, and how should they deal with their treatment and priorities?

Dr. C: You have to talk to your oncologist about your treatment schedule, number one, because you're still in control. Just because the oncologist wants to start next week doesn't mean you have to. We've already said that. Take your time. Get everything organized.

Everyone needs a really good support team, so you need that in your personal life while you go through cancer and you need it at your business. You really might want to think about two kinds of teams.

Rearrange your schedule, so you only work half the day. You're not going to be debilitated just because you're going through cancer. You can still function pretty well, especially if you have support for your health and wellbeing.

Most people have a couple of bad days where they feel really exhausted and toxic right after they get their chemo, but that's not every day, so plan for that. Look at your chemo schedule. When you're going through radiation therapy, usually you can function most of the day. You might want to think about scheduling your appointments, so they work for you, not so they work for the radiology center. Make it work for you.

There's a category we haven't talked about, which is the person who lives with cancer as a chronic illness. Those are stage 3 and 4 patients who still have some disease burden but are going to live a very long time, so they need to pace themselves. Most entrepreneurs drank the Kool-Aid and are accustomed to 60- and 80-hour workweeks. Doing that does not allow health, so you have to rethink what's reasonable to have health.

Most people in the age demographic where cancer is diagnosed have children or loved ones they really care about and want to be around for. I like to remind them that nobody ever says on their deathbed, "I wish I spent more time working." People say, "I wish I spent more time with my loved ones."

An entrepreneur is in control of their schedule, is in control of what they delegate and what they don't delegate, so it's an opportunity to use that. If you're bootstrapped to your new business, then it's an opportunity to see what is not essential for you to do and what you could actually give away or train somebody else to do, so that you have time for your self-care.

When you're going through the active phase of treatment, it's a part-time job, so you need to free up about 20 hours a week to take care of yourself, so you can get really well. You need a couple of hours every day for yourself. You need enough rest. You need to not sit in front of a computer all day long. You need time to eat, be healthy, take your herbs and supplements, be at ease, and have the opportunity for your nervous system to be in a relaxed state. That's a learning curve. Lifestyle and behavior change are the most challenging parts.

In my clinic I have a nutrition and lifestyle coach that works with my patients to help them implement all of these things, which is not easy. You can take advantage of that kind of support where you might have someone helping you with lifestyle and behavioral changes: how to organize a new diet, how to organize your supplements, and how to think through it.

Working with a health coach is a really great solution because habits die hard. If we also have been rewarded for the way we've been doing things because our business was successful and we made a bunch of money, then we might be loathe to change those habits, but it's absolutely possible to do that.

Get pragmatic. That's my one-phrase solution: be really practical. Most people are baby-steppers, not quantum leapers (even though we all want to be quantum leapers). Figure out a few small things you could change this week. Be successful at doing that. Then go to the next ones. That's where a good coach comes in.

MK: For someone who's going through surgery, chemotherapy, and radiation, what are the most common side effects? How you can treat them safely without interfering with the chemo and radiation?

Dr. C: Think about the cancer journey in phases, and each phase of your journey has its own unique needs. There's the phase when you first get diagnosed. The first trauma is the diagnosis. The next phase is when you're in treatment. Then the next phase is when you're recovering from your treatment. After that, either you're going to be living "life after cancer," with the goal of not having a recurrence, or living with cancer as a chronic illness. That's the journey.

Inside the treatment phase are subphases, like chemo,

radiation, surgery. Each one of those needs to be addressed uniquely.

There are a couple of extremely common side effects that all cancer patients experience. The most common side effect is fatigue. About 95% of cancer patients complain of fatigue during and after treatment. Some cancer patients and survivors complain of fatigue for up to 10 years after successful treatment, even when they have no evidence of disease.

This also applies to "chemo brain" or what we call "cognitive impairment." Both cancer and cancer treatment actually affect the structure and function of your brain. For an entrepreneur, your ability to think clearly, make executive decisions, analyze information, listen, and remember, all of those things are extremely important.

What's the common denominator? The common denominator is inflammation, so we want to have a plan to control inflammation. Now, cancer itself is an inflammatory syndrome, and the treatments are inflammatory, as well.

We can eat an anti-inflammatory diet. Number one, that means removing all refined, chemical, and hormone-laden foods from the diet. It means eating a plant-based diet that's rich in color. It means removing foods that are triggers of inflammation. It means including many more healthy fats and oils than what you might think about in a culture that said fats are bad. That looks like olive oil, almonds, almond butter, avocados, hummus, tahini. Things like that are very important to include every day.

Half your plate is colorful, organic, chemical-free vegetables, fresh, not packaged. Then a quarter of your plate looks like healthy, clean protein. Then 1/8 of the calories on your plate will be these healthy fats and oils. Notice there's no grain or carbs on that plate.

About the protein, you want to have adequate protein as part of your plate. You need about 60 grams of protein a day to maintain the energy you need during treatment and to maintain your muscle mass. Losing your muscle is part of cancer physiology and part of inflammation, so you really need to protect that. If you're not eating enough protein, you're not going to be able to do that. I use a shake as an insurance policy in a lot of my plans so that on the days when you don't feel like eating, you're not interested in food, or you're just busy because you're an entrepreneur, you have an insurance policy to get this nutrient density.

Another principle of cancer control is to lower your blood sugar and lower the hormone insulin, which is a response to eating carbohydrates. This means removing from your diet any starches and sweets. That might be grains. That might be potatoes. That might be fruit and sweeteners.

We also want to remove the artificial sweeteners because they are just chemicals. A chemical-free diet is essential to the cancer patient because most cancer patients are inefficient detoxifiers. That's part of being vulnerable to cancer. The first thing you do is just take all the packaged foods out of your diet. You remove a huge amount of chemicals and eat fresh, colorful, whole unprocessed foods.

It's not so hard to do today. Even if you live in a place where there aren't natural food stores, there's the internet, so there's places like Thrive Market, where you can get natural foods at very reasonable prices delivered to you. Go to the farmers' markets, things like that.

Then we can add anti-inflammatory herbs and supplements. I think about a foundation plan of nutrition.

Then on top of that, there's a second tier of the targeted things for your cancer environment, your cancer terrain. You want to have a multivitamin that has the active forms of all of the vitamins and minerals and that is copper-free and iron-free because copper and iron drive cancer growth. Then you want to have some omega-3 fatty acids, which are the EPA, DHA fish oils. If you're vegan, there are vegan alternatives to that. You want to have a good probiotic or eat plenty of fermented foods in your diet because your gut and the healthy bacteria in your gut influence inflammation control, detoxification, immunity, neurotransmitters, and a healthy brain, so that's incredibly important.

Most cancer patients, especially those going through treatment, need more magnesium, so you want a nice, highly absorbable form of magnesium, like magnesium glycinate. Then you want to have vitamin D3. Those are the core nutrients that you need.

A lot of the cancer treatments affect your nerves. Why does that happen? Because a lot of cancer treatments produce what we call a lot of "oxidative stress." That means that there's a lot of free electrons running around that are bouncing around damaging your cells. You need something to quench that. That's where we come back to our plate that is full of color.

If you just eat the rainbow, you're going to have a lot more antioxidants in your diet. That's like spinach, kale, carrots, butternut squash, persimmons, blueberries, pomegranates, things that are really deep in color. As long as your diet has a lot of color and you're picking mostly vegetables and only berries for your fruit, then you're going to have super antioxidants in your diet. If you don't think you're going to eat a lot of plants, then in that shake, I put greens powders and reds powders. That's my insurance policy if you don't eat all your vegetables every day. It can be simple. It can be doable for a busy person.

Let me add too that most patients do tolerate shakes and nuts. Patients with colorectal cancers or who have had radiation or surgery to their lower digestive tract will have difficulties digesting certain things like you did, but that's not true of everyone. People find out what works for them.

If you've had chemotherapy for any reason, your microbiome and your healthy gut bacteria have been wiped out, so you really have to work on that. Part of my training is Chinese medicine. In Chinese medicine, we say, "Saving the earth is the very first goal." What that means is save the digestion. Think about it. If your digestive tract doesn't work, all these healthy foods, nutrients, and herbs we're giving you, you're not going to be able to utilize them. It's absolutely essential that take care of optimizing your digestive function and restoring a healthy microbiome.

A good nutritionist or functional medicine doctor can help you do that, but at the very least, eat fermented foods (if you're not dairy sensitive). You can do yogurt and kefir. You could do healthy sauerkraut or kimchi, fermented vegetables. In Japanese food, there's a lot of fermented foods like miso and natto. Almost every traditional diet has some fermented foods in it, but it's easier to take a good probiotic.

You can't restore your gut if you don't also have healthy fiber in there. It's very important to be eating enough plant fibers so that all those healthy bacteria you ingest can flourish. If you don't build up your flora in there, it doesn't matter how many pills you take of probiotics. You have to have enough fiber in there from your diet for them to establish and colonize. That's very important.

One of the side effects of chemotherapy and radiation is that your blood cell counts may be depleted. Some chemotherapy agents actually wipe out your bone marrow function. The bone marrow is the factory for your blood cells. Some people misunderstand their anemia and think they have iron deficiency anemia, but the anemia, the low red blood cells from cancer treatment, is not about iron. It's that the bone marrow factory has been damaged. Acupuncture and certain Chinese herb formulas are my preferred way of restoring the bone marrow, but exercise and rest help to restore your bone marrow and your immunity, as well.

It's very important to make sure that you restore your muscle mass if you have lost some of your muscle mass. This has to do with managing inflammation, which we just spoke about.

Another way to manage inflammation is to take omega-3 fish oils or a vegetarian source of omegas. Also, the plant chemical curcumin, which comes from the turmeric root, is very important in naturopathic oncology. Curcumin interacts with over a hundred different genes. There is absolutely no drug that does that. Curcumin is something you could take for the rest of your life. One of its functions is to support normal inflammation and to restore the brain. The blood-brain barrier is damaged by cancer and cancer treatments, so healing it is important.

The other thing to consider is what's happened to your liver from toxic therapies. You want to be able to make sure you take into account the extra work the liver's had to do under toxic therapies and to restore it. A very simple way to do that is to add green drinks to your daily protocol. That might mean celery, spinach, lettuce, and lemon all put in a Vitamix together, something like that, or greens powder.

Also the American herb milk thistle can be taken in extract or powder form. If you're doing a shake, you can put it right in your shake, or you can put it in a cup of hot water or ginger tea. Take about a teaspoon twice a day during your recovery period and really clear out your liver, reduce liver inflammation, and restore liver function.

MK: You talked briefly about exercise. A common thing that I see happen in people, and I did this as well, is I got scared, so I started working out too much to try to make up for lost time. But once treatments kicked in I was completely fatigued.

How much is too much exercise? Can you trust your body to tell you when too much is too much, or should you push yourself? At what point should you just quit exercising because it's not doing anything for you? What should the regimen be?

Dr. C: Let's talk about the psychology of entrepreneurs for a minute. Entrepreneurs think more is better quite often. They are people who have the capacity to work even when they're tired and to keep pushing through because that's what makes a successful entrepreneur. However, it might not make a successful cancer recovery.

We have to look at our personal traits and qualities that might've made us successful in one part of our life and ask if that particular trait is useful or not in terms of recovery and treatment.

The first answer is the middle path.

The second answer is listen to your body. Our minds can trick us, but our bodies are pretty reliable sources of feedback. If you're tired, rest.

The most important thing is don't overtrain, middle path. Studies show that moderate exercise during and after cancer treatment improves outcomes. You do not want to be sedentary, but on the days right after chemo or if you just had a big surgery, you need to sleep all day, so you have to be appropriate. This is the cultivation of wisdom and discrimination, and really listening to your body.

A lot of entrepreneurs have the quality too of what we call "delayed gratification," meaning you can put things aside in order to do something unpleasant. This is a time to integrate and to not dissociate from the wise feedback that comes from your own body. Instead, really listen.

This is an integrative, developmental journey in this way. You're going to be in a body you don't recognize, so you must listen. You're going to be going through something non-ordinary for a period of time, so you have to be adaptive and do what's appropriate.

Generally after surgery and after an infusion of chemotherapy, you need to rest. I don't actually want you to rest all day. I'd like you to go out for four 15-minute walks, if that's all you can do. You shouldn't be still all day because one of the risks of cancer and cancer treatments is blood clots, so you absolutely do not want to be sedentary all day long. You need to move. Think about it. You want your kidneys and liver to filter, you want to expel CO_2 from your lungs, so you must move. You want your heart to beat, so your blood is moving. It does not serve you to not move.

If you had a certain level of fitness and exercise that was normal for you before your treatment, then you can begin to approximate that. Remember, you're in a body you don't recognize anymore, so you have to see what this new body is going to tolerate.

If you're also anemic because you lost a lot of red blood cells due to surgery or treatment side effects, then you're not going to have enough oxygen to push yourself physically the way you might be accustomed to. The key is to listen. In our culture, people are rather disembodied and disconnected from their bodies, so we don't listen. Do you know if you're thirsty? Do you know if you're hungry? Do you know if you're tired? Do you know if you need to stop exercising?

This cultivation of really listening and getting connected and being empowered to know what you need, that's really the bottom line because there's no recipe for everybody.

If you were more fit when you started, you can be more active as you go through it. The research shows that a minimum of 30 minutes of vigorous walking daily changes outcomes. Now, almost anybody could do that. Almost anybody could take a 30-minute walk. If you could only take two 15-minute walks, then do that. This is not a time to push. This is a time to be balanced and understand what you need.

MK: How do you recommend managing the communications and negotiations between a patient who either is 100% for or against an integrative approach and their spouse who has a different value system?

Dr. C: I'll actually tell you a story that happened just yesterday. I had a medical doctor come to me who is a cancer patient. She comes from a family of medical doctors. There's massive pressure on her from her family—her husband, her father, her sister-in-law who are all physicians—for her to do what's called "standard of care." "Cookbook medicine" in oncology is huge. She, herself, is much more interested in a balanced approach. She wants to include a health model, but more, she wants individualized care.

We were talking about whether or not she should do a therapy that's standard for women who have estrogen-driven breast cancers. The conversation we had is appropriate for most anyone making medical decisions. We asked, "What's the risk? What's the benefit?" If the risk is more than the benefit, I say, "Let's think about it." If the benefit is more than the risk, I say, "Let's just manage the risks, side effects, and the downside."

In her case, I felt that the risk was higher than the benefit of the therapy that was being recommended to her. I also said to her that the reason that physicians don't treat their family members is because they can't make neutral recommendations because they're emotionally hooked in.

A medical family will have a lot of fear if the patient doesn't do the standard of care. The patient themselves might have a lot of fear if they don't do the recipe. The very best thing to do is have individualized decision-making.

In research, there is this phrase called "N of 1 or N of 20." The N means how many people are in a study. There's a philosophy in integrative oncology where every single cancer patient is an N of 1. Every single cancer patient is unique and should be looked at that way. Why? Because a tumor cell line is unique. The one in you is different than the one in your neighbor, even though you have the same diagnosis. Those cells are different. They're occurring in your body, with your genetics, lifestyle, and diet.

Because of all that, an oncologist and someone like myself should say, "Okay, let's look at this, let's actually look at the data, let's actually see whether or not the standard of care makes sense for you. If it does, let's do it. Let's manage it. Let's get that great result. If it doesn't, if it's actually not in your best interest, you better put the brakes on, ponder, think, analyze, test, and do whatever it is you need to do to make a decision that's about you." That's the best way to go forward.

The other thing is most family members and friends who love you are going to go into overdrive because of their own anxiety. There has to be a time when you say to all these people that love you, "I know everything you're doing is because you love me, but it's now no longer helping me. Now it's causing me duress, and the greatest thing that you could do for me if you love me is to respect my values and my wishes. After you have said the same thing to me three times, I've heard you. You do not need to say it again. I've heard you." Then you have to really make a boundary.

Be patient and try to understand who can be there for you and who cannot. Some people will freak out and be so frightened about cancer itself that they can't be part of your support system. Some people will be able to be with you wherever you're at, support you, listen to you, and not get their own personal stuff all mixed up in it.

It requires having a spine if you're going to think for yourself and put together a plan that feels congruent for you but that might be a little outside the box. You need to ask the people who love you to do what loving is, which is to respect you, honor you, and respect your differences.

The other thing is healthcare is an extremely personal choice. What feels right for you might not feel right for your wife. Let's say she made a decision for herself that you wouldn't have made for yourself. You have to respect that because we're all adults here. We each have the right to make our own choices about our own bodies and lives. That might not be the dynamic in your family system, so it's time to address it if it comes up.

MK: You've got a variety of resources, services, and programs. Why don't you talk a little bit about those?

Dr. C: My book is called *32 Ways to OutSmart Cancer: How to Create a Body Where Cancer Cannot Thrive*. It's available on Amazon. My book gives you, as a patient or a family member, a way to begin to look at the things that make the most difference in creating a physiology that's not supportive of the development, progression, or recurrence of cancer. It is an accessible resource. It has 32 things you can do, in terms of diet, lifestyle, personal care products, exercise, a lot of the things we talked about, as well as some of the most important foods and safe herbs that you could take. It's a great place to start.

I also have a website that was designed for families, patients, caregivers, and supporters at www.IntegrativeCancerAnswers.com where there's a lot of free information that expands upon the things we've spoken about today.

I have actually 4 downloadable PDFs on that site that speak to the different phases of the cancer journey—if you were just diagnosed, you're in treatment, you're recovering, or you're moving on to live a healthy life after cancer. I have summaries of things you should be thinking about, how to talk to your oncologist, and what's important during that phase.

There are several hundred recipes on that site and several hundred blog posts about things that are of concern to cancer patients and survivors. Those are all complimentary resources for healthcare professionals, especially the frontline healthcare professional of all persuasions.

I have an online professional training available at www.AIIOre.com, the American Institute of Integrative Oncology Research and Education, which I founded to teach my "outsmart cancer system." The reason for this is that I can't do it all, and there's a huge number of patients who have no one to turn to for the support of their health during and after their cancer journey.

If you're a clinician who feels that there's a gap in your learning and you feel insecure and not confident in assessing these patients and knowing how to guide and really support them, then this is a 24/7 online training in which I also have live mentoring so that you can ask your questions, present your cases, and really build your skills, so that you do feel comfortable. Half the people in my course are medical doctors.

Everyone really feels the pain of not having this knowledge and education because if you didn't actually specialize in oncology, you're not prepared for this rising tide of patients that are living a long time after cancer, like yourself, who need support and monitoring to feel confident that they are doing everything possible to be healthy. I always say to patients, "I don't want to have the cancer conversation with you again." I don't want to be with a patient a second time talking about cancer and cancer treatment, so how are we going to get there? How are we going to have a health model? How are we going to have health experts? We can train clinicians, but how are patients going to find them?

That's sort of my mission right now—to leave a legacy after 35 years of practice. I'm thrilled to be talking about this with you because I think it's also a paradigm shift for a cancer patient to think about beyond the oncologist what they can do and where their resource people are going to be.

Entrepreneurs typically have a team of people that support them in their business. You can take your professional skills and habits, and transfer them to your personal life to look at your health as another one of your projects and manage it just like that. Take your skill set, your experience being successful, and apply it to your health.

MK: To wrap up, are there any passing words you want to share?

Dr. C: The most important thing to really understand is that you're in control of what happens to you. You may not know what to do, but you know how to find resource people. That's your first job: to make sure you have a team and to understand that you are going to be at the fulcrum of how this journey goes and where it goes.

Always remember that each person that you are seeking advice from must absolutely listen to you deeply, understand what's important to you, and respond to that. If you're in a care provider's office where that's not happening, find somebody else to be your care provider and keep asking questions. Cancer is a fascinating world where there's new information every day, so if you have access to a newsletter like mine or if you're a care provider and you want to be on the leading edge, then there's always more to do.

When I started in practice, we had no research on herbs and vitamins. We had traditional medicine. Now we have modern medicine, where I can say, "I could give you an herb to turn on a cancer suppressor gene." I couldn't tell you that 30 years ago.

Find the resource people that are going to stick with you through your longevity, through your health. Your oncologist is going to be done with you after a finite period of time, but your health team is going to stay with you for the long haul. Find out who that is.

Let me also say that you, Mike, are an extraordinary role model. You don't know it because your daily life is normal to you, but you're the exceptional patient. If your listeners and readers want to know what that looks like, the kind of person that gets to be an outlier, the kind of a person who gets to have this exceptional outcome, then they can look to you.

You were a stage 3 colorectal cancer patient. Your risk of recurrence is high. If you can accomplish this and transform yourself into a healthy person, healthier than before you were diagnosed, you're the role model for what it takes to do that. People listening and reading need to pay attention to what is actually required, so you're a very inspirational role model who is not painting a rosy picture. It's hard, but it's, of course, worth it. It's really important to have role models like you.

Please note: the transcript of this interview has been edited.

Survivor Interview: Hal Elrod

MK: Hal, why don't you tell people, very briefly, who you are and what you do?

Hal Elrod: My name is Hal Elrod. My wife is Ursula Elrod. We've got two awesome kids, Halston, who is 5 years old, and Sophie, who is 8 years old. That's my family and my number one.

I am the author of a book called *The Miracle Morning* and creator of *The Miracle Morning* book series, which has roughly 10 books in it. I'm a keynote speaker. Those are my main two things. I do a little bit of coaching and put on live events every year.

MK: How did you find out you had cancer, and what happened next?

HE: After I gave a speech in Colorado, I was walking through the airport to my gate. I was out of breath, and my first thought was "Shit. Am I this out of shape? I know I haven't been exercising very much the last few weeks, but am I this out of shape I can't even walk through the airport without being winded?"

The next night, I woke up in the middle of the night struggling to breathe. Just gasping for air. I didn't know what the heck was wrong. When I stood up the next day, it got real bad, so my wife sent me to urgent care. They said, "I think you have pneumonia." But they weren't very confident in that, so they said, "Get a second opinion if it doesn't get better in a couple of days."

A couple of days later, I still couldn't breathe, I was sleeping sitting up in bed. When I visited the doctor, he found out that my lung was collapsed from fluid building up outside it from my lymph nodes being enlarged.

Over the next 11 days, I had my lung drained with a giant needle. They stuck it through the back of my rib, and they would drain a liter of fluid at a time. Picture one of those giant Fiji water bottles, I mean a liter of fluid. They did that every other day for 11 days.

Then I learned that I had acute lymphoblastic leukemia, which is one of the rarest and most aggressive forms of cancer. In fact, it also had a cellular mutation to where they said the closest they could give me was a 10% chance of living.

MK: When you found out, what were your first concerns?

HE: When my doctor called me in, he said, "Hal, one of two things is happening here, you've either got some sort of unexplainable virus in your chest that's causing your lymph nodes to expand, or you could have some form of lymphoma, some form of cancer."

At the time, I'd been living an anticancer lifestyle for going on 10 years. Ten years earlier back in 2005, I watched a documentary called *Healing Cancer from Inside Out* and learned about all the dietary causes that can create tumors and cause cancer, and how to live a lifestyle to where, either if you have cancer, here's how you can kind of beat it, and if you don't have cancer, this way of living should keep you safe. I was living that lifestyle. We had no chemicals in our house. We were as natural as we could possibly be.

So when the doctor said that to me, I was thinking, "There's no way it's cancer. There's no way it's cancer. There's got to be some sort of infection."

Also I had just fallen in the lake and gotten a concussion, just a few weeks before. I swallowed a lot of water. They had had a sewage spill on the lake, and I thought that might have created some sort of infection.

I left though, and I started thinking, "Okay, anything is possible, who knows what this is?"

The first call I made was to my wife, Ursula. She and our children had gone on a trip to visit my grandma in Colorado. I got very emotional because I was thinking how she was going to receive this news. I know her well enough to know that she would have the fear, "I could lose my husband. I could lose the father of my children. Hal could die."

I knew her mind would go to the worst fear. I knew how hard that would be for her. I broke down crying on the phone with her not because of where I was, but because of where she would be. I tried to assure her, "Sweetie, everything's going to be okay. Let's not even think it's cancer until we know it's cancer, if it is. It's probably not. It's probably an infection, I'll probably be fine."

I waited to call my parents, and next I actually called my business partner, one of my best friends, Jon Berghoff. I said, "Buddy, this is kind of crazy, but remember how I had that breathing problem ..."

He knew I couldn't breathe, and he was worried for me. All my friends knew. I had to cancel a speaking engagement during those 11 days I was not able to breathe, so he was at a loss for words about how to respond when I said it might be cancer.

"Jon," I said, "You know me, I live by the 5-minute rule." That's something I learned about 20 years earlier from a car accident. I was hit head-on by a drunk driver when I was 20 years old. I broke 11 bones. I died for 6 minutes. When I came out of a coma 6 days later, I was told by doctors I would never walk again. Everyone ended up thinking I was in denial because I was so happy all the time, even at the doctors' words.

The reason I was happy, and I apply the same thing when I had the cancer diagnosis, is I accept all things I can't change. There's no value in wishing I could change something that is out of my control. If I have cancer, I have cancer. If I get hit by a car, if I lose whatever it is— acceptance is the key to unlocking the door to emotional freedom. All of our emotions that are negative are self-imposed, they're self-created by our level of resistance to our reality.

I decided 20 years ago, I'm not going to ever resist anything that I can't change. I'm going to accept it fully. By the way, that doesn't mean that you're happy with it. I wasn't happy that I might have cancer, but what I was ended up much more powerful than happiness.

Imagine over on the right side we've got all the positive emotions like happiness, love, and joy. On the left side, we've got all the negative emotions like fear, anger, resentment, and sadness. In between on this emotional spectrum is a place that I call peace. It's rooted. You could be happy one minute, and a phone call makes you angry or depressed, right? Emotions are fleeting, but when you accept all things you can't change, you live in a place of unwavering, unconditional peace. From that place, you're grounded to where you can choose whatever emotions serve you in the circumstances.

I told Jon, "If I have cancer, I can't change it. I won't feel bad for a second. I'll feel bad for my family anytime I think about what they're going through because that hurts me that they're hurting. But me, personally, I'm at peace with that. Look, the car accident that I was in, I view as the best thing that ever happened to me because it made me into the person that I am today. It gave me a purpose in life, a story, and a mission that I can serve humanity in a bigger way."

I told Jon, "I don't even know if it's cancer, but if it is cancer, I believe this will be the best thing that ever happened to me. This will be part of my evolution. There's some sort of lesson that I am meant to share with the world."

I don't know what it is, but there's no negativity towards this experience. I'm going to embrace it, I'm going to learn from it, I'm going to grow from it. And on the other side of it, I will beat it. I have unwavering faith that I will, and I will be a better version of the person that you know today.

That was it. That was my response. And it was the response that I chose for the entire journey, which is "I can't change that I'm immense pain right now because of some procedure or some infection, but I can be at peace with it as much as possible."

MK: In Louise Hay's book *You Can Heal Your Life* she gives the emotional causes of disease. Her belief system is that we all create the reality we live in and that there are emotional causes for the diseases we get.

Do you believe there was an emotional or spiritual cause of the disease for you?

HE: I'm a huge believer in the mind-body connection. There's a lot of science that shows our thoughts, our mindset influences our biology. We can literally change our DNA. We can write all of that. I believe that in a practical sense because I experienced it already with that car accident.

When the doctors first called my parents in after I was out of the coma for a week, they told my parents, "Hal's in denial because he's always happy and smiling." They thought I couldn't accept what was happening to me, so I was in lala land, but it was the exact opposite of that. I had fully accepted what happened to me. I was genuinely able to choose to be grateful and to be happy.

A week later, the doctors came in with routine X-rays and said, "We don't know how to explain this, but Hal's body is healing so quickly that actually we're changing our prognosis from 'he's never going to walk again' to 'he can walk tomorrow.'"

Three weeks after the crash, they took me into therapy in a wheelchair, and I took my first three steps. It was all I could do, and I sat back down.

Earlier, I'd told my dad that if I'm in a wheelchair the rest of my life, that I will be the happiest person you've ever seen in a wheelchair. But I also said that's only one possibility. The other possibility is that the doctors are wrong, and I will walk again. I said, "That's the possibility that I want, so that's the one that I am visualizing every day, I'm praying about it, I'm talking about it, and thinking about it, I'm feeling it in every fiber of my being—walking again. I'm feeling my legs move again."

Fast forward to the cancer diagnosis. There's a few things. I accepted the worst-case scenario that I might have cancer, and then I did have cancer. Then I accepted the worst-case scenario that I could pass away, and if I do, I'm at peace with that. However, that's not what I want. What I want is to be completely healed and to live to be 100.

All my cancer affirmations ended with #2080, because that's the year I'll turn 101. I literally have that affirmation where I visualize my daughter at my 100th birthday, she'll be 71. My son will be 68. Their kids will probably be in their 40s, and so on. My great, great grandkids will be just about 10 years old. I visualize being a happy, healthy 100 years old. Then I bring it back and visualize having hair again (that I did get back and it's kind of curly like yours too).

I'm bringing this back full circle to what may have caused my cancer or what I believe. I actually read that Louise Hay book. The emotional cause that she pinpointed for leukemia did not resonate with what I had. I kind of dismissed that in a way.

But I don't dismiss the concept that our biology is impacted, influenced, and even determined by our psychology. Because of that, I did ask myself the question "What may I have done to cause the cancer?" even though we will likely never have conclusive clarity on why it happened.

The doctors don't even know what caused it. Their theory was that I had a lot of radiation when I had my car accident. They think that radiation 20 years earlier could get stored in my DNA and manipulate my cells. Then when I got my concussion three weeks before I was diagnosed with cancer (I ended up having to go in for a CT scan and an MRI), they think that might have activated these dormant cancer cells, so that's a theory of theirs.

But guess what? I don't have any control over that, so what I wanted was actionable changes that I could make. I wanted to look at how was I not living that perfect, healthy life. I was living healthy, but I wasn't perfect. I had vices. When I was tired, I didn't choose rest, which is what your body's telling you it needs when you're tired. I chose coffee because I value productivity above rest. That was one of the causes that I wrote down that might be a cause of cancer and something that I have control over that I can take actions to improve moving forward.

Whether it caused cancer or not, it could have, it could have not, but it was something that wasn't ideal, so I needed to value rest and taking care of my body above productivity or whatever else.

Another big one was I had been diagnosed with ADHD when I was 25 and prescribed Adderall. I've taken it off and on in very small doses, which is how I'd justify it to myself: "It's so small, I'm taking 1/10th of what they're prescribing me." Then I'd quit, then I'd take it for 6 months, and then I'd stop taking it for 6 months. It's been this off-and-on journey. I realized that might have caused it.

I wrote an affirmation to remind myself: "I will never ever, ever, ever, again in my life take Adderall." I supported that with the whys: it could have caused my cancer; therefore, taking it literally could remove me from the lives of my children and my wife, and that is unacceptable. I will never ever risk my family's well-being for me to be more productive.

I identified these areas. The last one I'll share, and a friend reminded me of this. He said, "Hal, do you remember about 6 months ago, when I was visiting you, you told me that there's this unconscious belief that would occasionally become conscious in you? It was that you thought you didn't deserve the success that you had and that some sort of major adversity must be on the horizon because that's what your life's been like? It was the car crash, then the financial crisis, so you're kind of due for the next one? Remember how you told me you were thinking that?"

I had this limiting belief based on a lack of deservedness. I think of the Marianne Williamson quote, "Who am I to be special, fabulous, gorgeous, talented?" We all deal with that. That insecurity, that general self-image of "I'm no more special, I'm just me."

I had that. I was waiting for the next adversity unconsciously.

So again, I have an affirmation now that says, "I will never, ever again get cancer or any deadly disease because I deserve to live a long, happy, healthy life."

MK: Is there anything more that you want to add about your fears?

HE: Not being there for my family was really the only fear I had.

When I had my car accident, one of the big elements that I mention in my book about it is the moment that you accept responsibility for everything in your life. The degree that you accept responsibility for everything in your life is the degree that you have the power to change, improve, or create anything in your life. I think the big area there that people have a challenge with is the distinction between taking responsibility and blame.

I have a family friend who was hit by a drunk driver. It happened 20–30 years ago, and to this day, she hates that "son of a bitch." Every year on the anniversary of the day, she posts a scornful Facebook post saying she hopes he's "rotting in hell." She has so much blame.

To me, the difference between blame and responsibility is blame determines who's at fault, which is of the least amount of value. Great, who cares? It was someone else's fault, great.

Responsibility determines who's committed to changing things. Who's committed to healing? Who's committed to growing? Who's committed to improving? It doesn't matter who's at blame. All that matters is that we fully accept the responsibility for creating the circumstances we want in our life, despite whatever anyone did or whatever happened up until this point.

MK: Let's talk a little bit about the treatment you chose.

HE: I mentioned I watched that documentary, *Healing Cancer from Inside Out*. After watching that, my plan was to never do chemotherapy. If I ever got cancer, I would just go to a completely alkaline diet. I actually have a friend that went on completely alkaline diets, and she avoided chemotherapy because her tumor shrank and went away. She's been cancer-free. So that was always my plan.

When they said I might have cancer, I told my wife, "Sweetie, it's fine. We already know cancer cannot live in an alkaline environment, and yadda, yadda, yadda, so that's what we'll do." She says okay.

Then, we went in and got a third opinion at MD Anderson, one of the best cancer hospitals in the world, and from one of the top leukemia doctors in the world. My doctor is brought to leukemia conferences almost every month. He always somewhere in the world talking to other oncologists about the cutting-edge, latest technology and protocols. I felt I was in good hands.

I sat down with him the very first meeting and said, "Doctor, I'd like to build the body and heal the body with natural, holistic protocols. Can you support me in that?"

And he said, "Hal, you'll be dead in a few days to a few weeks."

I thought that was a scare tactic. I didn't really like that answer, like they're scaring me into chemo.

He repeats, "If you don't start chemo, you're going to be dead in a matter of a few days to a few weeks, maybe a week."

I said, "Okay, can I have 24 hours with my family? Go figure this out, discuss it?"

He said, "Yes, but I wouldn't wait longer than that."

We went home and we googled. We used Google. That actually should be a t-shirt: "Google ever cure anyone's cancer?" What we found was my cancer was so rare that if you googled my cancer, page 3 of Google was the first time you saw anything about it. It was specific, acute lymphoblastic leukemia. Then I had a cellular mutation that made it even more rare. It caused the cancer cells to radically duplicate, which is why I went from being totally healthy one week to almost dying with a failing kidney, collapsed lung, and heart failure a week later. It was so rapid, so quick.

One step further, I started reading this book by Suzanne Somers, who is big into holistic curing. She has one of the best holistic doctors in the world, Dr. Burzynski. He's out of Houston, which happen to be where I was at MD Anderson. He's Polish too, and my wife believes in anyone who's Polish. For her, it was divine intervention, so we're feeling like it's meant to be. We reached out and long story short, he basically said, "Your cancer is so rare there's nothing I can do for you."

I'm going, "Holy shit! If one of, if not the best holistic doctor in the world is telling me there's nothing he can do for me, I don't think enough google searches are going to solve my problems."

I was resistant, but I agreed to do chemo. We started chemo the next day, and the chemo regimen that I had was one, if not the most intense chemotherapies that you can go through. I've talked to other cancer patients, and they'll go into chemo for one day a month or one hour. Just my maintenance chemo is 15 minutes a month for 3 years.

This was 5 separate chemotherapy drugs, for 12 hours each, for 5 days, overnight in the hospital. Just one chemotherapy drug in my vein after another, after another, after another, after another.

What I ultimately decided to do was to include the best holistic practices I could find, basically as if I weren't doing chemotherapy. I wanted to build my immune system, detoxify my liver, and cure cancer.

My dad told me, "Hal, you don't need to be researching all this shit. You need to focus on healing and not stress yourself out. I'm going to put together a team of your friends, and me and your friends are going to do this for you."

He formed a team called the Healing Hal Team. They did all this research. They would look up cannabis, they'd look up everything. They would synthesize the information, bring it back to my dad, and talk it through. Then they would bring me what they felt was the most relevant information.

For me, it was a game changer. I was going through cancer, and there are days, weeks at a time, where you're unconscious. You're bedridden. You have no energy to talk, let alone research.

MK: It is incredibly grueling. It's my opinion that you made the right decision doing the integrative solution, but nuking it first. Look at you now, you look great. You're still thin, but you've always been a thin guy.

HE: Yes. I didn't have 40 pounds to lose when I lost them, but yes.

I want to just insert this before I forget, in case it doesn't come up again. There is a website called chrisbeatcancer.com. He is a pretty young gentleman, I think he's 33, and when he was roughly 20, he got stage 3 or stage 4 colon cancer, I believe. I'm doing my best to remember what it was. The doctor told him he would be dead in a matter of weeks or months. He prayed about it and decided to go 100% holistic, and he cured his cancer.

Then, he went on a journey to find others. He created a blog, and he's interviewed pretty much all of the world's best holistic doctors as well as dozens, if not hundreds, of people who cured their cancer naturally.

I've talked to him on the phone too. I love his heart, I trust his heart and the way he brings information to folks. I really appreciate him. I've even seen articles that he's gone back and reneged on something that one of the doctors said based on further findings. He's really diligent about bringing the most wisdom and truth that he possibly can. I highly recommend that as a resource.

MK: I've met him a couple of times and had pretty extensive conversations. I don't agree with everything he says because it's easy, from my perspective, for a really young, healthy person versus someone who is in their 50s, 60s, 70s, or 80s and who may have a slightly compromised system or maybe not the discipline to do all that it takes. That's why there is no one answer for this that' good.

HE: Here's the thing: my doctors don't know anything about anything, and these are the brilliant oncologists of the world. I would ask them, "What part does diet play in my healing?"

They would say, "It doesn't matter, just do the chemo."

I'm thinking, "What you put in your mouth matters no matter what. You can't tell me that."

And then I would say, "I've read up a lot on liver toxicity, and that sometimes people die from chemo. In fact, quite a few people die from chemo because the chemo builds up in their liver and it creates toxicity and it leaks into their body and they die. What can I do to detoxify my liver?"

They go, "Oh, don't worry, we give you a little flush after each chemo."

They know nothing about it because the pharmaceutical companies that fed the meds fund the meds said it was cool, right? With that, I realized that I'd have to do my own research.

After my second chemo, they tested me for leukemia, and they couldn't find any. So I went, "Oh, cool, let's stop doing the chemo then. You got it, right? We're done?"

They go, "No, our instruments aren't 100%. And as rare as your cancer is, if we stop it now, it will certainly come back stronger, and it will kill you."

I go, "When can I quit? When can I quit putting the poison that is chemo in my body?" That's how I was feeling.

Then I called you and your perspective was "Listen to you flippin' doctors! Do what your doctors say."

When I first got cancer, part of what inspired me in the very beginning was that I wanted to use it as a platform to write the book that frees people from thinking they need to go poison their body with chemo. That's what I was thinking.

Because I was so resistant, I wondered, "How soon can I quit chemo, so I can write a book about how I did it mostly natural?"

What I finally realized was that if I had written that book, I would have impacted very few people. Because if you're sitting across from the oncologist, and your family member or your spouse is next to you, and you say, "I know the doctor's saying that I'm going to die if I don't do his protocol, but I read this book by Hal Elrod. I know you haven't read the book, sweetie, but Hal's really trustworthy, so I want to do what he said," then nobody would listen to my advice. I wasn't going to listen to an author over the guy telling me I'm going to die.

What I realize is I was given an opportunity to go through the world's most difficult chemotherapy, or one of them, given a 10% chance to live, and then given an opportunity to combine the best of allopathic Western medicine with the best of holistic Eastern medicine, and do as much research as I could to make sure I wasn't interfering with one or the other. Because even the supplements that are great for you are bad for the chemo; they hurt you. I had to be really careful, really diligent, but like you told me: trust your doctors.

I will tell you, Mike, that one of the most important affirmations that I wrote for myself wasn't about why I might have cancer; it was about why I might die from cancer or have it come back.

It was later in the journey that I realized that I'd been hanging onto a new unconscious belief: my chemo could cause my cancer to come back. But that fear is gone as far as me thinking that I'd someday say to my wife and father, "I told you I should have stopped chemo early, now I'm going to die."

My solution for getting rid of that fear was to maintain 100% certainty, unwavering faith, that my Hyper-CVAD chemo was working perfectly and that my cancer will never ever, ever, ever come back.

I would remember how Tony Robbins' son Jairek got malaria in Africa, and he asked Tony if he should take a medication that he was prescribed at the hospital. Tony said, "I don't know anything about that medication, but whatever you choose, Jairek, have 100% certainty that it will work, and it will work."

That's the same 100% certainty, AKA unwavering faith, that I had to maintain during my chemotherapy. It goes back to that mind-body connection. I truly believe that if I had hung onto that resistance to the chemo and felt it was doing more damage than good, then it probably would have.

For me, it didn't get nearly as bad as it gets for most people that endure 1/10th of the chemotherapy that I endured. I believe that's because of the holistic support that I gave myself.

I detoxified the heck out of my liver. My doctor didn't tell me that I needed to. He didn't give me the information. I just googled, "How do you detoxify your liver?" I figured out milk thistle. Then I googled "Is there any conflict with chemotherapy and detoxifying with …" I went as deep as I could.

I did coffee enemas. I did all these things, what I call extraordinary effort, whatever I could do to detox my body and build my immune system in between my chemo treatments. I believe that's why I had it easier—I feel like I had it easier from stories I heard of people that would just go in for an hour a month of chemo versus my 5 days straight.

By the way, I just ran across this—it was Chris Wark, the "Chris beat cancer" guy. Something that really resonated with me. He says it's important to have peace about what you're doing, whether it's chemo or not. He's very religious; he says God heals in a lot of different ways. There are people that are healed that go through chemotherapy, there are people who are healed without it.

It really does need to be a prayerful, informed decision whether or not you're going to do chemo. You have to make that decision with your family.

If you are someone that was like me and you're resistant to doing the chemotherapy or whatever, be at peace with it. That has as much to do with anything.

As far as how bad it got—after I would get chemo, I would always have some minor nausea, a little bit of throwing up, but again, that's where I felt like it wasn't as bad as I'd envisioned it.

Part of that is actually allopathic medicine. There's a drug called Zofran. A friend who had gone through cancer said, "Zofran's a miracle." It keeps you from throwing up like crazy, so they give you that while you're getting the chemotherapy.

The worse that it got was I had to get 8 injections of chemotherapy in my spine. They're called "lumbar punctures." With my particular cancer, there were enough cases of people where it would travel up and hide in the spine. The chemo would kill it in the rest of the body, and it would go hide in the spine and then travel up the spine and turn into brain cancer. They told me they would prevent that by injecting chemotherapy into my spine. I'm going, "Hell no! You're giving me enough chemo!"

Then we did a little research on google, and actually we found there was a Facebook group for every kind of cancer, which is so important. It's great to have access to other people and their journeys. However, I would advise you to have someone in your life—a friend, a family member, caretaker, spouse—be the one that monitors the Facebook group.

My dad told me about the Facebook group, and then a day later he said, "Don't ever go in there. Hal, people are dying every day, and we don't need you to see that. Obviously, we know people are going to die from cancer, but you don't need to be exposed to that every day."

But it was helpful because he asked in a post, "Has anybody dealt with a lumbar puncture? How did those work?"

And this one woman said, "My husband refused the lumbar punctures, they got rid of the cancer, he was pronounced in remission, and then it traveled up his spine and he died of brain cancer."

I went, "Okay, I'm doing the lumbar punctures."

We'd been warned. I had to sign off that there were major potential complications of a lumbar puncture. It was a new nurse who did the lumbar puncture, but she did it crooked; she messed up on it. Within 24 hours, I had the worse migraine headaches I've ever had in my entire life, and I grew up with migraine headaches.

My entire life I've had migraine headaches once a month, maybe. I thought I knew what a migraine headache was. I had never experienced such horrific pain to where I couldn't handle any light. I could not handle a single sound. I had earplugs and white noise the whole time. I couldn't eat any food. It was 4 days in the hospital without eating a single bite of food because I couldn't keep anything down. I couldn't even open my eyes to eat food.

My poor father, who's my caretaker, he's just dying inside watching me go through it and not being able to help. I ended up staying 6 days in the hospital, and they finally kicked me out. They said, "We know you're in pain, but we need the room for chemo for somebody." They sent me home.

My dad and I had an apartment by the hospital. Twenty-four hours later, I'm in the fetal position. I haven't moved, haven't eaten. I think it was then, 6 days, and my dad's trying to give me broth. I'm lying there, and he's putting broth in my mouth. I'm just telling him, "Dad, stop talking, I love you, stop talking, I can't handle it."

Here's a game-changing lesson that I learned in the next 5 minutes. My dad said, "Hal, I know you don't smoke marijuana, but do you want to try that marijuana that your friend Brianna sent you?"

And I said, "I'll try anything, sure."

The funniest part is, my dad has never smoked marijuana, I don't believe, so I'm coaching him as I have my eyes closed on how to pack a bowl of marijuana, how much to put in. It was so funny.

Then my dad's holding up to my mouth a little glass pipe that my friend sent me. He's lighting the bowl, and here's the magic: I took 2 puffs.

Now keep in mind, I was on 7 prescription drugs at that point: one for pain, one for nausea, one for migraine specifically. I don't even remember what all the other ones were. They had me on 7 prescription medications for 6 days, and they did nothing except damage my liver from whatever toxicity was there.

Two hits of a plant that grows in the ground, that luckily is becoming more and more legal, and 5 minutes later, I was sitting up in bed (I've got pictures of this and a video of this). I was smiling, I was laughing, and I was saying, "Dad, I'm starving, make me a sandwich."

And I was simultaneously angry that there are 1.5 million cancer patients in the United States, to my knowledge, suffering as bad, if not worse than I was, and who are on all these prescription medications and many of those are not working for them, when something that is natural and grows in the ground is being withheld from them. It solved all of my problems in 5 minutes.

That's when I started diving deep into the research for cannabis. We dove deep into it, and I found a source where I could get it. I didn't want to smoke it because I didn't want to hurt my lungs, so I was able to get capsules. You're just taking the oil, and it's by the milligram. You can make it very specific.

Other low points in my journey: I had one chemotherapy cause horrific stomach aches for about a week and pains in my upper abdomen. They gave me all sorts of prescriptions. For a few days I was bedridden. I was in fetal position, I couldn't work, I couldn't do anything. This happened twice, one of these two chemo treatments that I took two different times.

I feel so strongly about it now that one day I might be lobbying Congress about legalizing marijuana, at least for medical use nationwide. Luckily it's state by state. It's been a game changer for dealing with symptoms.

There's some evidence that it can help cure cancer. I don't know that there's enough to count on that, but definitely to manage symptoms, it's a game changer. In fact my aunt was just diagnosed with breast cancer, unfortunately, a few weeks ago. I got her some. She's terrified because she thinks of marijuana like it's heroine or something. But I said, "I promise. Just a little bit, just take the capsule."

MK: In the midst of this, you've got a real business. You've got a real business partner. How did your cancer and your treatment affect your business? And how did you manage your business while you went through this? What team members were critical?

HE: Two things that I recommend every business owner entrepreneur puts at the top of their list is, first and foremost: building passive sources of income. That's number one.

For me, I've got 11 books. We both have right around 11 books. As you know, books are a passive source of income. So that, for me, was able to pay the bills while I was getting my cancer treatment.

Number one is to have passive sources of income, whether it comes from books, real estate, online courses or information products, or something hard, tangible.

And the second part is building a team.

For a few years I've been talking about the importance of building passive income. I wrote an article on entrepreneur.com, and I went as far as saying that it is selfish to *not* do that. Both being selfish toward your future self and selfish toward your family if you have one.

We can't count on one source of income, especially in today's economy. Millions of people are out of work because they were counting on that one source. Even as an entrepreneur, if you just have one business, one source, one thing, and it dries up all of a sudden, you're in trouble.

I believe that we have a responsibility to create as many streams of income as we can. You, Mike, are living this to the umpteenth degree.

Now I can tell you with a whole new perspective why that's important. Because one in two men, they say, is going to get cancer in their lifetime, and one in three women. That means half of us better have some extra income. Cancer is stressful enough, and if I didn't have that income coming in, it would have been a whole different journey. It would have been a stressful, fearful, horrible journey if I didn't have the bills paid because I wouldn't have known where the next paycheck was coming from.

I feel so much for people. In fact, we started a nonprofit called Support the Unsupported. And we're waiting for our 501C3 status. When I was in the hospital, I realized how many people didn't have the support that I had, both in terms of people, in terms of knowledge, and in terms of resources. I want to help folks that don't have that.

About building my team: I've got two business partners. Jon Berghoff and I run our live events and Masterminds together. And Honoree Corder, we are 50:50 partners on the *Miracle Morning* book series. I'm 50:50 partners with Jon Berghoff on the Mastermind and the live events, and with Honoree on the book series.

Honoree was able to keep the book series going all year long as if nothing ever happened. He just checked in with me as needed. I got cancer about a month before our live event that I had 300 people coming to. They were going largely to see me. Up until the day of my flight, that was actually that lumbar puncture that I got in my spine the day before I was supposed to go to San Diego for my event. Obviously, I had to cancel the event. I was able to stream in for about 20 minutes before it got really bad. Then after that, I was supposed to stream in every single day of the event for 3 days. The next two days there was no chance, and that was it.

Having business partners that could run the business while I was in the hospital was incredible. Jon Berghoff took over my podcast. He's still been running it for the last year.

And I have Tiffany, who's my director of operations, a personal assistant. She handled everything. She was me. All the communications, all the emails. She booked all my speaking, everything.

Having a rock-solid personal assistant that knows everything about the way you run your business is crucial. In fact, that's where I would start. Number one is you gotta hire that person.

Here's what I encourage people to do: if you are a newer entrepreneur, and you're going, "A, I don't have the capital to hire an assistant. B, I don't know how to hire an assistant or how to train them or what they would even do." Go on Amazon and find a book on how to hire an assistant. Google it.

Here's my advice: start with an intern. An intern is free.

Here's a great way to find your next assistant—I was at a restaurant, and this server, Tiffany, she was amazing. Her level of professionalism and the way that she was so attentive to us. I said to my wife, "She is a rockstar. I need someone like that as my assistant."

She goes, "Why don't you see if she's open to any other work?"

I went, "You're right." And I offered it.

Tiffany responded, "Actually, I need an internship."

In my head, I go, "So wait, work that I don't pay you for? That sounds like a good deal."

She was my intern for 4 months. Don't tell her, but I would pay her any amount of money, so she keeps doing what she's doing.

That's the main team that I've got.

MK: For me, during the worst of my treatments, when I was going through radiation and chemotherapy, I had about an hour of usable strength per day. And I had to do everything I could in that time.

What did you do? How much time did you have, and where did you spend it? When you did have time to spend on your business and the areas that were mission critical?

HE: For me, it wasn't really a daily thing. It was hard for me to not be able to schedule every day because I'm a very scheduled person. Every hour of every day I've got my schedule planned out. Because of my symptoms and the way it would go, I'd be in bed for 4 to 5 days.

It was kind of like the flu, you could say. Like where you can't think straight, you can't do anything, you're just exhausted. So, we'd just go through periods.

And then I would feel, actually, totally normal. In fact, the funny thing is while I was getting chemo, I felt amazing. The first time I went through 5 days of chemo, I felt guilty. I'm like, "I feel fine." I was working on my computer the whole time. I could work during the chemo.

Then I started to get a little fatigued. It was actually 10 days after my chemo that my counts would drop, and I would just hit my rock bottom. That would last anywhere from 4 to 7 days.

What was weird is it did a mind trick on you because you'd feel like, "I'm great, feeling great with chemo." Then after 2 days or after 5 days: "I'm feeling great. I guess this one wasn't so bad." And then you would just crash. It would hit 10 days later.

For me, I would just do the work that I would normally do. I work from home on my computer. It's mostly just answering emails, communicating with team members, and putting people in place to do what they need to do. I'm a keynote speaker, and I had 4 keynotes booked. They were 6 days apart in 4 different locations, two countries, three states. I also had a Paris keynote booked and an Italy trip booked during my cancer.

The 4 keynotes, I tried to reschedule them, but they really wanted me there. So, I finished chemo—and this is just a God thing that I was blessed with the right energy at the right time. I was weighing a 127 pounds, I'm 6 foot 1 and bald, and my dad was my caretaker. He flew with me. It was crazy. Thursday night we flew to Florida. I gave a keynote

Friday morning for Pure Romance, which is a group of 2,500 women that sell sex toys. You couldn't have asked for a more fun group to have my first keynote back. I got a standing ovation. I was so nervous.

You're nervous when you haven't spoken in a while, but I also added the fact that if they'd followed me for many years, they're probably wondering why I looked like that. And I didn't know—my keynote is so dialed in, how do I enter the cancer story? Do I put that in? I just decided that if it comes up, it comes up. I'm not going to plan it at all.

It ended up being at the very end of the speech. So the elephant in the room, which is me onstage, the way I look, it was like I was recapping the lesson I shared, that I talked about earlier, which is accepting all things you can't change.

I said, "You guys, this isn't just something I did when I was 20. I do it every day in traffic. I also did it 3 months ago when I was diagnosed with ..."

It was literally like I said 3 sentences at the end to wrap up the lesson I'd just taught them and bring it to the forefront and how I just used it.

Then we flew to Montreal, Canada, right after that speech. Then we flew to Phoenix, Arizona. Then we flew to Vegas. We did those 4 speeches.

So, I still was able to pull off those 4 keynotes. But, I had to cancel my London trip, which was a book tour. And I had to cancel my France keynote two days beforehand. And I was the headliner, the poster, the entire website, the event—and I felt so bad. Luckily they were awesome, and it is what it is.

MK: I get it. I had the same thing. I booked a speaking opportunity at a Tony Robbins event. I spoke at Business Mastery, and I accelerated my treatment, so I could be there. When I walked on stage, same thing—I'm almost bald, I weigh less at a 150 pounds, which was light for me. I look like a skinny little Auschwitz victim. And the crowd went wild. They just stood up. I just stood there and I cried.

HE: How could you talk?

MK: I couldn't. It was incredibly moving.

My last question: what was the best piece of advice you received from anyone about cancer?

HE: The best piece of advice I received about cancer was that I was in charge of my treatment, that I needed to make decisions and not let anybody bully me into doing anything that I wasn't comfortable doing.

Obviously that's a fine line to walk between trusting your doctors and all of that. But I'll give you an example: take responsibility for your care, no matter what you're doing in the moment. I would have doctors come in, for example, when I was neutropenic, which for anyone that's not familiar with that, that means that you have no white blood count, and, therefore, you have no immune system. If you get any sort of germ, you can die. You literally have no immune system, so they have to use antibiotics to fight it artificially.

So I would see doctors come in and nurses, and they wouldn't have gloves on. I'm not a very bold person in terms of I don't want to make people feel awkward. So my natural personality is just to kinda let things be. And nothing's a big deal.

But I really took ownership, and I went, "Sir, can you please put on gloves before you work with me? I'm neutropenic. I've been told that everyone should wear gloves."

And they'd go, "Oh yeah. Sorry."

So really take ownership of your care.

The other piece of advice that is equally the best is having a caretaker. It was having my dad there at those times when I was in so much pain that the doctors would come in and they're trying to diagnose me and I can't think, let alone talk. I'm barely overhearing my dad running down the events that have led up until that day in a way I could not have. I remember feeling so grateful that he was there for me because I couldn't do it myself.

MK: On the other side, what's the worst piece of advice you got from anyone, whether it's a person or a doctor, that you either did or didn't take?

HE: Real simple: it was my doctor saying that nothing natural mattered. I realized it's not their fault, they're great people, and they mean well. It's just that they don't know. All they know is what was in the textbooks, that they read and studied to pass the exams.

And from what I understand, a lot of that is created by pharmaceutical companies, so if they can't profit off of it, they're not really recommending it. It's a business. Hospitals, it's all a business. "Go eat a bunch of healthy food, that'll cure your cancer"—that doesn't work for their business. So, I have to keep that in mind, but also have that trust.

MK: They're also in the math business. They just look at the data. They've got patients going through there who say they're living a healthy lifestyle. But again, if you go to Jamba Juice, a Jamba has twice as much sugar as a can of soda. So someone might think that having 3 Jambas a day is going to help their cancer. And it's like, "Nah." And you can get into a whole thing: refined sugar or fruit sugar and everything else. The net is, they're in the math business.

HE: If there's a best piece of advice, it's that the most important thing to take ownership of is the end result. You have to own that you are going to make it. That you are going to beat it.

I believe in the mind-body connection. You can do your own research on the mind-body connection. But that's one thing from every book I read on people that have healed themselves of cancer—whether it was done allopathically or naturally or a blend of both—is that all the doctors that observed them said every person that beat cancer had already decided in their mind that there was no other option and that they were going to beat cancer.

And so I encourage you to create a mantra for when you're going through those tough times. Write it in the form of an affirmation, so you read it every day: "I am committed to healing cancer, and I'm going to beat cancer." In your own words, but there is no other option. And whenever you're having doubt, read that. And read it with conviction: "There is no other option. I'm going to be at my hundredth birthday party."

MK: Where you are right now? You're mostly in maintenance mode at this point for all practical purposes, right?

HE: Yeah, I just did my first maintenance the other day.

MK: Is there something that you wish you would have done differently that would've made your treatment or your experience easier or better?

HE: The resistance to allopathic medicine is probably the one thing that if I would do it again I wouldn't have any resistance. Luckily after a few months I got there.

But for those few months, it was a real stressful time for me internally. And also stressful for my dad because he saw the stress that I had and that I was resisting it. It caused him to resist it because he didn't want to see me go through chemo.

The other one is cannabis. Again, luckily I figured that out within a few months. But it would have saved me the most horrific 4 days of my life, pain-wise. And then there were some other times where it would have really helped me.

I wish I would have known about the cannabis, and I wish I would have just not resisted the treatment. Just embraced it. You helped me to do that by the way. So, thank you.

MK: That's great.

You've touched on it, but I'm going to ask the direct question: whether it's mentally, spiritually, business, family, or your own personal journey, what do think the greatest gift from your cancer has been?

HE: The greatest gift has been that my family will get a better person. My kids will have a better dad. And my wife a better husband.

I'm a workaholic. I was probably in denial about that. Of course, I worked just for the family. I'd justify the little time I did spend with the family by saying to myself, "That's more than most dads do."

Here's the reality: most of us say that family, or the people in our lives, are number one. The question I have been asking people lately is "Does your schedule reflect that?" If you looked at your schedule and it's like mine was with 95% of your time spent working and 5% is with your family at the end of the day, what's leftover of you when you're exhausted and angry and grumpy—is that really giving your family the best of you, if they're the best of your life?

I made a lot of decisions in the hospital and away. I lived half of this year in an apartment by the hospital, not with my family at all, which was hard. My kids literally were growing up without me. And there was a real disconnect. We're still working through getting them back to trusting me. Because it's like, "Mom, mom, mom, mom, mom." They're so dependent on mom because I was gone so much. It's almost like the negative effects of me being a workaholic before the cancer were amplified 10 times over by me being out of their life completely. I wasn't even at home.

When I got home, the first Saturday that I was home, my son came downstairs. He's my little miracle morning buddy, he's my early-riser. He said, "Dad, are you going to come down?"

I said, "Halston, we can do anything you want today, it's Saturday. We could go to the zoo, we could go do racecars, we could go to the park. We can do anything you want. What do you want to do?"

He said, "I want to go play with my action figures in my bedroom."

I said, "Buddy, okay, we can do that, but we could do anything." And I named all these cool things.

He goes, "I just want to play with you in my bedroom and my action figures."

In that moment, I realized that's his favorite thing to do in the world. That means more to him than anything, and how freaking hard is that?

So I said, "Buddy, how would you like to do that every single day before you go to school, before I take you to school?" And he just lights up.

I said, "Give me a second." And I pulled out my phone, and I typed in "30 minutes of playtime" from 7:45 to 8:15 every single morning. Now me and Halston, my son, do that every morning.

At the end of the day, my daughter and I hang out—it's in the schedule, 5:00 to 5:30, as soon as I get off of work.

My wife and I put our kids to bed together now. It used to all be my wife, as in, "You take them to school and I'm the provider. You take them to school, you pick them up." I now take the kids to school every single morning, one of the two. It's family.

I think the greatest gift that led to that, that I can impart with anyone reading this, the greatest thing that I could share is the question that I've been asking that led to that answer, which is, "What matters most?" And those three words may be the most important words in the world. I ask them in the big picture, but then I drill it down and go: what matters most to me being the father my kids deserve? What matters most for me to be the husband that my wife deserves? What matters most in my business and it running while minimizing stress?

I've let people go out of my business that were causing me stress. I've limited travel, I've reconfigured a lot of things, things I didn't like doing.

I was running a group coaching program for the last 6 years, and I just announced, right in the middle of my cancer journey, "Hey, this is the last year, we're done." I just did my last call, we have one more call this month, so now we're moving on.

"What matters most?" I believe is the question that you've gotta ask every day of your life. Be really clear about it, and then the follow-up question has to be "What do I need to do to make sure I'm living in alignment with what matters most to me?"

Please note: the transcript of this interview has been edited.

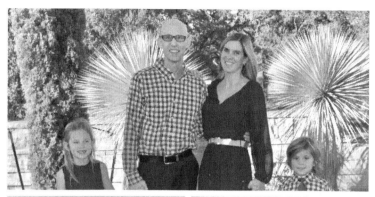

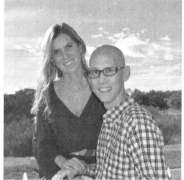

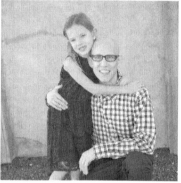

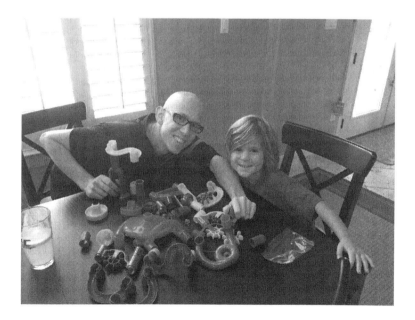

Survivor Interview: David Wagner

I met David shortly after meeting my wife and we had an immediate connection. He grew up very close to me in a small rural community in Minnesota. He worked in the "hair" business, was very entrepreneurial and shares my warped sense of humor that requires be raised with no money, in a small town, powered by hope and irreverent. My wife and I helped in launch and promote his book, "Life as a Daymaker", built his first web site and then watched him go through cancer...as an entrepreneur. Looking back, I didn't realize until writing this how profoundly David's experience affected me. He shares some fantastic wisdom in this interview - and I hope you enjoy the video too!

Mike Koenigs: David, why don't you share a bit about you and your background?

David Wagner: I became a hairdresser at the age of 18. I decided not to go to college and went to beauty school instead, much to the chagrin of my dad. I was lucky enough to start with Horst Rechelbacher in his first school, in the first class. He was the founder of Aveda. I started with him. I went to Europe for a couple of years and trained with some of the masters there and then ended up coming back.

I started applying some of my experience to the salons at Horst. He had just started Aveda and needed people to run the organization, so I became vice president at the age of 23. I had a blast doing that. Then I started my own company, my own salon when I was 26. I ended up going back and merging with Horst 3 years later when I was 29.

A year later I bought him out. Now we have 10 salons in Minnesota, one in Palo Alto, California. We just bought a new company down in Arizona 2 years ago. We have 13 salons total, 500 staff. We serve 400,000 guests a year.

I think what made our business is our being a "daymaker." What that means is we purposefully make somebody's day. It's like saving a woman's life by simply being kind as a hairdresser. I ended up writing a book about that. It became a bestseller. After that, all of a sudden not only our organization was known for it, but other industries and platforms have taken over being daymakers as well. I'm really proud of not only our company, but what it stands for: *daymaking*.

I wanted to be a dad when my kids were much younger, so my wife and I moved to Maui, Hawaii, and pretty much set Juut up to sort of run itself (I'm a huge fan of Michael Gerber's *The E-Myth* series).

What I learned years ago was working *on* the business, not *in* it. I consciously started to try to work on my business versus in it. I found that when I was in Maui away from the day-to-day, I was able to get away from the static. I was able to think more creatively and think about fewer things, but in bigger ways. I could think about 5 years out versus the problem of the day or putting out the fire that just occurred.

I brought in a great team that led Juut, and I was in Maui for 7 years working on the business. I filled the steward of our brand and worked with the president and the directors of the salon.

That's when I discovered that I had cancer. I was away, but it was still going to affect my business because I wasn't sure in what capacity I'd be able to work on the business, much less in it.

MK: How did you find out you had cancer, and what were your first thoughts or concerns?

DW: I was in Maui. I was working with a personal trainer and trying to gain more flexibility. I was having some pain in my hip. First I thought I had piriformis, so I was doing stretches for that. Then I thought it was sciatica. He started doing some work on me and said, "Why don't you go get an X-ray?

I want to make sure that you don't have a hip spur or a bone spur in your hip."

I got an X-ray. In Maui, the medical facilities are pretty lacking. The diagnostic place was next to Denny's. I got my X-ray, and a few hours later, I went back and picked it up. I was sitting in my car in the parking lot, and I was just curious.

I pulled the X-ray out and put it on my windshield. I noticed that one of my hips was fully white, and on the other side it was different. I pulled the radiologist report out, and it said, "Bone cancer, likely caused by prostate cancer, lung cancer, or that it metastasized from something else."

Here I was sitting in the Denny's parking lot by myself reading this diagnosis from someone that I had never met. I didn't know what to do.

So, I went to my doctor in Maui. Picture this: his office is in a yurt in the rainforest. I drive up to his yurt. He puts the X-ray up against the window. He just turns white.

He was a friend of mine. He said, "God, David, I don't know what to tell you. This doesn't look good. I'm going to set you up for some bone density tests and a blood test."

Then I talked to my wife and shared with her the report. I downplayed it because I didn't want to scare her. I thought, "If it's bone cancer, maybe I can just have it cut out or they can do something to regenerate the bone."

I was deceiving myself too. I was really trying to not make a bigger deal of it than it was.

When I went to get my bone density test and a blood test, my doctor couldn't get the results because he wasn't an orthopedic person. Another friend of ours from our kid's school said, "I'll get the test for you."

When he saw the results, he called me and said, "David, you have to go back to the mainland. We can't treat you here." He thought that I had multiple myeloma. I didn't know what that was. It's a blood disease.

I went back to Minneapolis a few days later, and the kids and Charlie, my wife, stayed in Maui because I didn't want to scare them.

In Minneapolis I called in some favors, trying to get the best doctors that I could. I was at home by myself when they called to tell me the results of the tests. It an assistant to the doctor. one that I had never met who called and said, "We just wanted to let you know that you have multiple myeloma. We don't treat that, but we'll refer you to another oncologist that is a specialist."

No information, no prognosis, nothing. I, of course, get online and look up "multiple myeloma." It has a 3-year life expectancy. I'm like, "Fuck." On one hand, I felt really fortunate because I had 3 years. I knew it wasn't a couple of weeks or a couple of months. I had 3 years.
My daughters at that time were 10 and 12, and I thought, "At least they'll be 15 and 13, right?"

For about a week I sat with that. When I called Charlie, I didn't tell her what I had because I knew she would google it. Then she and the girls came to Minnesota from Maui on spring break, if you can imagine, and never went back for a year.

When they arrived, I continued to decline. I ended up losing 35 pounds, ended up in a walker, and then ended up in a wheelchair. When I went in to have more tests for multiple myeloma, they did some bone marrow draws and more biopsies. They said, "It's not multiple myeloma."

I was like, "What?"

They thought I had something else, and they wanted to put me on treatment the next day.

I said, "I want a second opinion."

They said, "You don't have time for a second opinion." I was really in the worst shape of my life.

The president of our company, her husband works for this financial firm. He worked with this guy whose father was the head of hematology at Mayo Clinic. I was trying to get into Mayo Clinic, and I had an appointment in 2 weeks to see them.

What they told me at this other hospital was "You don't have 2 weeks. You need to start right now."

That day, the guy emailed his father and said, "There's this guy who's trying to get in early to Mayo. Can you help him?"

In the meantime, a friend of mine in Santa Fe knew somebody in Oklahoma that was the head of a lymphoma research foundation; lymphoma is also a blood disease. He said, "If I were you, I would either go to Sloan Kettering or Mayo Clinic in Rochester, Minnesota. But if I had one choice, I would go to Mayo, and I would see Dr. Habermann. He's the best in the world."

I said, "God, I would not only like to get in earlier, I would like to see Dr. Habermann." I had called to see Habermann earlier and tried getting an appointment with him, but they laughed it off like he's like this God.

My phone rings about 5 minutes later and I answer. I hear, "Hi, this is Dr. Habermann. I understand you need to see me. How about tomorrow at 1 pm?"

So many of the experiences that I had with doctors was "turn and burn." I felt like I was at county hospitals.

But the Mayo Clinic was amazing. Dr. Habermann had all my slides and everything sent from the other hospital. We sat in his office from 1 until 5 pm. Dr. Habermann came and went, and he had pathologists looking at all my slides.

He said, "This is complex. I hate to say it, but we're going to need another biopsy." He called a surgery team in and had a biopsy done that night.

The next morning he told us, "We know what it is." It was stage 4 large cell B lymphoma, non-Hodgkin's lymphoma.

When they did the PET, I lit up like a Christmas tree. I had tumors coming off every lymph node. It was in my bones and my marrow. That's why I couldn't walk. I had all these tumors that were invading every space of my body.

Dr. Habermann told me, "We'll start your chemo tomorrow." If I had more time and if it wasn't so severe, I would have looked into more alternative options, but I was going to die.

I did go to our naturopath. He did some energy testing on me and said, "Your body is going to love chemo." He gave me a couple of supplements to help me with the chemo or to help the chemo help me in a sense. He said, "I want you to start taking 10,000 IUs of vitamin D3." I started doing that.

Going through chemo is a really tough thing. You don't want to build your body up with nutrients because you're trying to allow the chemo to kill the cancer. If you try to build your body up in some regards, you're also building the cancer cells up. It's this weird dance of getting low enough that it can kill the cancer cells, but you want to be sustained yourself.

It's this who-do-you-believe game because everybody that I met, everybody that I knew, especially in Maui, had a cure and had a thing that I should be taking. I just gave myself up to Western medicine and said, "Okay, I'm going to take vitamin D3, but otherwise I'm going to turn my body over to you guys."

MK: Historically, the oncologist will say, "No supplements at all." Your oncologist was okay with you taking vitamin D3?

DW: He asked what I was taking, and I said, "The only thing I'm taking right now is vitamin D3." He didn't say to take it, he didn't say not to take it. I felt like he had something to say, but didn't say it.

About 3 months later he said, "When you told me you were taking vitamin D3, you might have noticed that I didn't tell you not to take it. In fact, I've been having this study up for lymphoma patients and outcomes. It's been specifically on vitamin D3. We just released the paper, and you're right on track. Outcomes for people that have significant amounts of D3 in their systems, those outcomes are 80% better." Now that's what they're recommending, but at the time they didn't have the paper.

My naturopath was right on. I trusted him and believed him, and then I wasn't talked out of it by my oncologist. In fact, he didn't encourage it until he could confirm it, but then once he completed his paper, he said, "You know, this will be what they recommend for everybody from now on."

Concerning the path of your treatment, I think you have to use your intuition. I don't necessarily recommend it to everybody, but one of the things in losing 35 pounds, I felt like my body was really depleted, going through the chemo especially. Charlie was talking with this woman who provides raw milk to people, and it's illegal in Minnesota to do that because of all the health concern around bacteria, but I intuitively felt like I needed it. I needed that kind of wholeness and enzymes and all of that stuff. Fortunately, we knew and trusted the farmer.

The reason I don't recommend people to just do raw milk is I don't know their farmer. You have to be able to use your intuition in some regards and be safe. I talk about it with people that are interested, but it's not that I necessarily urge them to go do the same because I can't control the quality of the raw milk they're getting.

MK: What were all the treatments you had and how long did it take? What were the short-term effects? The long-term effects?

DW: I ended up having R-CHOP. R stands for one drug, C stands for another drug. It's a cocktail for non-Hodgkin's lymphoma, or my specific lymphoma. The first time I had it 2 days to drip because the body has to get used to it. I'll never forget the first day when they said, "If you feel at all ... you'll be getting the shakes or tremors, just hit the emergency button."

All of a sudden, I started feeling that way, and before I could reach the emergency button, I was in full Keith Richards mode. I was just in this epileptic thing, and then the guy came in, shot the drip off, shot me full of Demerol to reverse the side effects. It literally took 2 days to receive the first dose of chemotherapy.

From then on, I went in every 3 weeks. It would take about 4 or 5 hours because the body was more used to it. Honestly, what my naturopath said, "You're body is going to love chemo,' was true. I had some slight nausea, but I went into the hospital the first time in a wheelchair, literally had to be wheeled in to get my treatment. The next day or 2 days later, I wasn't pain-free, but I could walk out of the hospital because my tumors had shrunk enough, and I felt relief. For 4 weeks before that, I kept going downhill, but all of a sudden after chemo, I had this bright spot of relief.

I'd thought I was going to even get lower. About a week later, the body reacts, and then I hit the wall. For a week, I felt fine, for another week I hit the wall, then the next week I start feeling better, and then it's time to get back in and get another dose. I ended up going through 9 doses, it took about 6 months.

After the fifth one, they do another PET scan, and they expect it to be gone and the final 4 to clean up. After my fifth treatment, I still had a hotspot in my pelvic area to show that it was cancer. They were really disappointed that they didn't get it. I went through another 4 treatments. Then they waited 3 weeks and did another PET scan. It still showed that it was hot.

This was a week before Christmas. They brought in a social worker. Because I needed to have a stem cell transplant, they were curious how we wanted to handle. I was going to be 90 days in isolation. Did the family need housing or what was going to go on?

I was like, "Oh my God." I'd been feeling better, but now I was going to have a stem cell transplant. Shit, it doesn't get much worse than that.

My doctor said, "You know, I want to do a biopsy and just make sure." I went in for a biopsy to make sure that it was cancerous. I had so many tumors that had shrunk and become scar tissue that they had to open me up.

A couple days later, it was Christmas Eve. My doctor told me, "I've got some really great news. What the PET scan was picking up on is abnormal cell growth. Typically, it's cancer growing. In your case, it's cancer dying off. It's still creating scar tissue. It's called narcosis."

The PET scan had picked up a rapid dying off of the cells, not a rapid growth of those cancer cells.

He said, "Merry Christmas, you're cancer-free." Oh my God, that was my Christmas gift.

MK: That's unbelievable. Now, at that point, had your bones started regenerating too? Talk a little bit about the process of recovery. From diagnosis to Christmas to recovery, what happened?

DW: My parents live near the Mayo Clinic. I decided to stay at their house the night before I first went to Mayo so that we'd be only a couple hours away. My parents lost a daughter when she was 13. She had a heart defect, and she ended up having a heart attack.

I did not want to bring that kind of pain and sorrow on them again. As much as I was concerned about my own life, I was concerned about them being worried about it. I decided to try to be inclusive and have them help me. My wife drove me to their house, and I got out of the car. I had a hard time walking. They literally had one step up to their door, the 6-inch step. I couldn't get up. My dad and my wife had to literally lift me into the house. My mom just started balling. That was about the worst that it could get.

I was able to hide it a bit from my daughters. They were young enough, and fortunately, cancer didn't mean dying to them because both their grandmas had breast cancer. We've known a few people that had cancer and recovered from it. Having cancer didn't mean that you were going to die. They knew that I was sick, but they weren't worrying about it in that context, but my mom and dad were in a whole different place. I tried to show a good face for them. It was just really difficult.

To be honest, I was trying to have a poker face, but I had no idea. I really didn't know if I was going to come out of it especially before I had the first treatment. It got so worse, and I just couldn't see pulling out of it.

MK: From diagnosis to you're cancer-free, how much time was that?

DW: It was 9 months.

MK: That was pretty fast actually.

That's the 9 months, but then it's been 8 years now. How long did it take for you to be able to move and feel normal again? When did you start noticing the change where your body started regenerating bone and you felt normal again?

DW: I was really lucky. It was probably after my first chemo when I felt like I could move.

I was fortunate to have Master Chunyi Lin here in Minnesota. I had seen him speak before and had done some classes with him. I went to see him 3 times a week and ended up doing Qigong. I had healings from him 3 times a week, and then I did Qigong about 2 hours a day. I had a massage therapist coming over once a week. People were bringing great food and all that.

As soon as I had my first chemo, and I started feeling physically better, I started working on getting stronger with my body. I started gaining weight back, and I was fortunate that I'd hit the bottom right before I had my first chemo.

I got better when I had chemo, which is rare. My appetite was stronger. It was this bizarre thing that my body really adapted to chemo.

MK: That's amazing. I think you're the only person I know of who's had that.

It's 8 years later. Do you still have some residual side effects that are noticeable? Where are you in your recovery?

DW: I find that I have to do pilates because I've got so much scar tissue in my core, my pelvic area, and my shoulders. It's pretty hard to bust that up. My flexibility really took a toll. I work 3 times a week doing pilates. I try to be as active as I can. I try to maintain my weight and eating.

Then I focus on my core—having some flexibility and busting through that scar tissue. It's not easy, it's pretty rough stuff too when I remember looking at the PET scans literally lit up like Christmas trees. I've got these pockets of scar tissue all over the place. When I get a massage or when I move my body in a particular way, I know it's there, I can tell it's there.

The thing that I had a hard time with was that it's in the first 2 years when it's most likely to come back. Every 3 months, I had to go back in for scans and blood tests.

For 2 months, I felt great. Then a month before I would go in for my scan, every little pain I thought was tumor growing again. When my hip hurt, I figured it must be back. I go in and it's like hitting my lottery every 3 months. Then you're fine for 2 months, and then you get this mind fuck that every little pain means it's back again.

The first couple of years, in particular, I committed to myself that I was going to do everything I could to not have it come back. Then after the 2 years, it was going every 6 months. After 5 years now, I go annually. Now I have 11 good months and then a month before, I have to go in for my annual. All these little pains, and I'm sure it's back. Every runny nose, and I'm sure it's back. It's this mind fuck.

One of the things that helped me see that I had light at the end of the tunnel was a friend of mine. She's in her 80s now. She was a client of mine since I was in my 20s. I used to cut her hair. She's about 30 years older than me. We became very good friends, and she sent me a note saying, "David, I know you're going to get through this. This is just giving you credibility for what's next." Man, I just hung on to that.

I had this photographer friend of mine come in and follow me on my journey. We did photoshoots. I had this really great slideshow basically of my journey. Then he went to Mayo with me a couple of times.

Now looking back on it, God, it just seems surreal. I did speaking, and I'd show some of those slides and the taste of the chemo would come back when I saw them. Even the taste of the Prednisone. I'd just get a stomach ache looking at the slides. This was 8 years ago. Yeah, *Mind Fuck* is the book I was working on then.

MK: Let's talk about business. What were your concerns? What were your fears? What was reality? What wasn't reality?

DW: As soon as your hair falls out in the hair business, it's the worst.

My first thing was to get a core group. I had 5 leaders that I brought into the loop. As soon as I got home, I had them to my house. I let them know that I had some disease, and the doctors were still working on it. I didn't want to tell them what I had until I knew what I had.

They agreed that they would step up in any way they could. As soon as I got my diagnosis, then I shared with them what it was. I don't remember sharing that I had stage 4. Non-Hodgkin's lymphoma is curable, but when it gets to stage 4, it's a whole other deal.

I told them what I had, but I didn't tell them the degree that I had it, which gave them some peace of mind that I could get through it. I didn't want to cause them concern where they wouldn't need to be.

The couple of people that I had closest to me that brought me to the appointment before Charlie and the girls got to Minnesota were scared to death. They saw how degenerated I was.

For others, I'd sit in a chair and talk to them. Sitting down, how sick I was wasn't so apparent, but watching me get in and out of cars—one of my leaders who saw that just didn't know how to handle it. She was my go-to person.

Looking back on it now, she and I are tighter than ever because we went through that together. She literally sat in the appointments with me at the doctor's office because Charlie was still in Maui. That's when one of your co-workers becomes such a trusted friend.

When I shared it with our staff in general, I was asking for their support. I was asking for their prayers. I let them know that if I wasn't getting back to them, it was because I was focusing on myself and it's probably going to take me 9 months to a year to heal. I have a great relationship with them. They were really supportive.

One of the things that my oncologist at Mayo said was "I know you've got a great business. People are going to support you. Watch out for ruthless competitors. I see this happen all the time. It's unbelievable." He sees a lot of high-profile entrepreneurs.

I said, "No way. Who would take advantage of me in this case?"

It blew me away how many people covertly were soliciting staff and making shit up about my demise. It was bizarre. It gave me this strength of showing myself and being really transparent.

With the help of my photographer friend that was taking photos of me, I made it really public. I shared my journey, talked about it, and was really open. I was trying to be as upbeat as I could, but still be transparent.

It ended up nobody left. It showed me who was who in our community here in the hairdressing world and who was willing to take advantage of it. It blew me away.

We became big supporters of this group called Angel Foundation, which supports non-medical costs for people going through cancer. I was flat out on my back for 6 months. I don't know how people could work even 10 hours a week going through what I did. I had a hard time getting up and eating 3 times a day, much less going to work and providing for my family.

I had the means to be able to focus on myself and not have the stress financially and all that. God, what most people go through and having to choose between their own health and livelihood or to give up their house. It's mind-boggling. I counted my blessings every day, and now I try to support those that are going through similar things that don't have the means.

MK: Let's talk a bit more about the business side. With the amount of limited time, energy, and focus you had, what did you spend your time focusing on in your business?

DW: I found that with the limited time that I had, I wanted to spend that on what gave me the most pleasure. That is designing creativity. It wasn't personnel issues, it wasn't expansion, it wasn't spending time with the finance department. It was designing.

I decided to open a new salon while I was going through chemo. I had the support of our facilities people, but I wanted to design it.

I went through design magazines. I was online looking at new stores that were opening in London. My mind was working in a really creative way, and it was giving me energy. It wasn't depleting. It gave me a reason to be up and stay up during the day.

I remember standing in front of my team, we had all 500 people in a room. It was a couple of months after I started chemo. I said, "My doctor asked me, 'What gives you the most pleasure?' and I said, 'My people.' Then he asked, 'What gives you the most pain?' I said, 'My people.' For some of you, I'm going to recall your calls and you'll hear from me, but the majority of you, I'm not going to deal with your bullshit."

Everybody started laughing. They knew exactly what I was talking about because it was all this petty shit, and I just didn't want to have my day consumed with that. Other people dealt with it, and more importantly, staff held it back. Even from my people they held it back because they knew at some point or in some regards, any complaint was going to affect my ability to thrive.

Our staff really stepped up in that way. They became problem-solvers themselves, looking for solutions versus pointing out problems. Having that kind of transparency with staff was really refreshing. Then being able to spend time on design and creativity and what's next, that was inspiring and uplifting to me, not a drudgery.

In fact, we opened that salon in the fall 6 months after I had chemo. It was a blast that I was able to envision something, bring it to life, and everybody rallied around it.

MK: When you actually returned, were you able to sustain that no-bullshit mindset?

DW: I'm a typical Taurus where I observe things and I don't respond, but I always keep it in the back of my head. I'll just listen and take it in, and then a month later I'll snap. It seems over nothing, but it's this cumulative effect. I knew that I was holding some of that stress and some of that angst in me.

What I promised myself when I got well was that I was going to tell the truth faster. When somebody would say something, propose something, or be critical, I just spoke my truth.

Now my people have come to recognize that I'm not being offensive or critical; I'm alleviating that angst and that energy from sitting in my body. We have these great debates and discord around something, but it's immediate, I don't hold it in.

I think my people are learning all that for themselves too: that it's okay to go toe-to-toe and come to a resolution faster. That's been the one change.

I used to be all listening, inclusive, and looking for all kinds of input. Now I push back a lot sooner and a lot quicker. I think people at first were surprised by it, but they know that I'm telling them the truth.

MK: From your point of view, including a genetic component, environmental component, or even emotional component, what do you believe caused your cancer? How did it manifest?

DW: From a linear point of view, when they said I had multiple myeloma and other people had died of that, one of the things was hair dying. I've been a hairdresser since '77. Some of the hair dyes that were suspect to that weren't taken off the market until the early '80s. That's where my head got wrapped around with multiple myeloma.

With non-Hodgkin's lymphoma it's typically a long-term low-grade infection or inflammation that causes that. For me, I had an abscess tooth in my 20s right in the front. I do a lot of speaking, it would flare up, it would go down, I'd go on antibiotics, it would relieve itself, but it always was lingering as a low-grade infection. My dentist kept saying, "We should pull it. You're going to have to wear a flipper for 6 months before we do the implant."

I just never wanted to do it. The warning that they give you for that kind of infection is heart disease because it can go into the blood. It's a low-grade infection that can cause heart disease. It can also cause lymphoma.

After I was diagnosed with lymphoma, I went in and had a 360-degree X-ray of my mouth. I had 4 pockets of that low-grade infection. As soon as I got through my last chemo and my blood count was high enough to have my teeth extracted, I had 4 teeth taken out.

When I had my first chemo, I felt, "Ah, that's relief." When I had my 4 teeth taken out, my body, it was like the same thing: "Ah, thank God."

It took me 9 months to get implants and have the bone heal and all of that, but that's what I felt was the cause of it from a physical point of view.

From more of an emotional point of view, I think that me being susceptible to it was my central nervous system.

I have this antenna that's really reactive. I can read people, I take everybody's shit on. I absorb too much. That's why I tell the truth more often now.

My central nervous system became compromised. Because my blood was compromised, I think that's what exacerbated it. I pay attention now not only to inflammation and cancer-causing foods and things like that, but also thoughts and my central nervous system being inflamed as well.

I think that I've got this wild radar. I've got this antenna that's really reactive. Now I tend to point it toward positive things versus reading negative things.

I'm engaged with politics right now. I'm watching all the bullshit going on, but if I get consumed by it, I'd be causing inflammation in my thoughts and all that. I try to be as positive as I can and just pray for good outcomes. Not being too engaged or involved.

MK: What do you think some of the best gifts of cancer were to you as a spiritual being, as a father, as a husband, as a business owner, or to yourself?

DW: When I was 26, I was involved in a minor plane crash that seemed like it was going to be a major plane crash. I thought I was going to die. We were coming to the runway, and all of a sudden I had this unbelievable sense of calm contentedness with what I had done in life. I wasn't married, I didn't have kids, but I had this contented feeling that I had done as much as I wanted to or could or whatever, that I didn't waste 26 years. When we landed and we were okay, I couldn't believe that feeling.

At the depth of my illness, I felt the same way where I truly didn't know if I didn't want to stay, but I was okay leaving. Having that conversation with my wife, I wanted to determine how I was going to leave if I was going.

Again, this contented feeling came over me, as in—wow, the reason that we spent 7 years in Maui was so that I could spend time with my kids. The universe was looking out for me and giving me all this time because of what I was going to miss or what they were going to miss going forward.

I felt how lucky I was, how fortunate I was, what a life I had led and the experiences that I had, so I was okay going. I was going to fight like hell to stay around, but at the same time, I was at peace. That was probably my biggest surprise from an emotional point of view.

Then being told that you're cancer-free, there's again this survivor's mind fuck too, like, "Oh my God, now what am I going to do with the rest of my life because all these other people that I know didn't make it?" I felt as daunted with the gift that I was given as I'd been about the situation that I'd been in. It was easier to go through cancer than going through the rest of my life.

I'll never forget, I had been planning my 50th birthday party in Maui. My birthday is in April, I was diagnosed in March. So, my 50th birthday party was at Mayo getting my first chemo. It's not the way that I wanted to spend my 50th birthday.

I often come back to this reality: you go in to get your chemo and there are 20 people waiting for their turn and how many 5-, 6-, 7-year-olds there are. You think, "God, I'm 50. I've had this full life. I've had all these experiences. How is it fair that these little kids are going through the same thing?"

I tried to use my experience as if going through a gauntlet. I tried to observe as much as I could so that I could share it with others. I'm still digesting it.

On one hand it's like I didn't even go through it. It seemed so surreal. On the other hand, it's like it was yesterday.

I have mixed emotions around the spirituality of it. I think I was prepared spiritually to leave.

I learned something from Master Chunyi Lin. I did this butterfly meditation twice a day that he does where he talks about not fighting cancer, it's not a battle. When you're in a battle and you're trying to kill something, you're exerting all this energy to kill. In his meditation he talks about cancer not being bad energy; it's just too much energy. That's the way spiritually I look at it too. It is this energy in my body.

It's called the butterfly meditation, and I would recommend it to anybody. You imagine the cancer cells leaving your body as butterflies blessing the world. Not that you're going to kill it or that you're in this battle or you're in this fight because that takes too much energy.

It's actually inspiring and uplifting and regenerative when you think of releasing these cells out into the universe as beauty versus killing something. That helped me immensely.

We've got friends whose 26-year-old son is going through it. I got him a recording of the butterfly mediation, and I said, "Think about this differently. Don't be in a battle because it takes so much energy to be in a battle. Heal yourself."

He isn't esoteric, but it gave him some relief that he didn't have to have this front with everybody that he's fighting a battle with cancer.

It's like the whole "fuck cancer" thing. I totally understand it. On the other hand, if you can look at cancer as a blessing, a wake-up call, and see all that you're going to learn from it, even if it means passing. It was part of my journey.

I have these conversations with very few people because it might seem selfish, but these were the realizations that I had. Why not me? This is part of my journey, and if it's going to be, I want to learn as much as I can on the way out. I want to impart as much wisdom as I can on my way out and now that I'm not on my way out, now what am I going to impart? It's just trying to live in beauty no matter which direction you're going to go.

MK: It really comes down to the power of reframing because that's what it is. It's a language pattern. You listen to the powerful language that someone uses when they're describing something. That's what's going on inside the brain. You're creating the inflammation and that stress response.

DW: Even being told that I was "in remission." I told my doctor, "I'm cancer-free." Being "in remission" means that it's still there, but it's dormant just waiting to wake up. That may be the technical word for it, but I consider myself "cancer-free," which is a lot less work.

MK: What advice do you have for someone who just found out they are diagnosed with cancer?

DW: Surround yourself with people that have resources, not opinions. I was so fortunate to be pointed to Mayo Clinic. I was fortunate to be pointed to Master Lin.

I must have 3 dozen books on fighting cancer. Everybody thought they would send me a book that they'd heard of. That's not it.

It's really about discerning who you're going to link up with, who you can trust to get to the care that you want. I think getting outside of the norm, not just going to who you're directed to, but really rallying your network around not what they think you should do, but who they think you should see because everybody knows somebody.

Get a couple of opinions. I saw 3 different people who offered 3 different routes to follow. If I'd followed the second one, I'd be dead. They would have given me the wrong cocktail. Fortunately, I persisted and pushed, and the universe worked out for me.

The other is if you've got the time, do the research. But you may not have the time. Mine was aggressive. Everybody wanted to send me to Thailand or Mexico, but I didn't have time. Then they were like, "Oh my God, he's surrendering to allopathic or Western medicine." But, it's okay.

Find the absolute best people you can that resonate with you and do not just get directed to somebody.

I think my advice about not fighting cancer, but trying to embrace the experience and look at it as too much energy versus bad energy, I think is the best advice that I could get.

MK: Master Chunyi Lin taught you the butterfly meditation and Qigong. Are there any other resources or tools that either helped you throughout the process or you've found about since and are using right now in your second life?

DW: There's a great book called *Nature's Cancer-Fighting Foods*. It's not that I only eat those things, but I'm now aware of what beats cancer, what diminishes cancer, what's anti-inflammatory, what's low in sugar, things like that. I didn't change my diet radically, but I avoid certain foods.

Even going through chemo it is important to pay attention to foods that feed substances, like even alcohol with sugar in it, things that cause inflammation or irritation. It is a good idea to find a nutritionist or somebody that knows food preparation that can teach you 10 different anticancer dishes. They don't need to be bland or macrobiotic or even vegan. It's like the "dirty dozen" with pesticides; there's a "dirty dozen" for cancer.

Becoming acquainted with that is really sustainable and to know that you're feeding yourself in a way that is suppressing or at least not waking up cancer is really smart.

MK: Are there any other final thoughts that you want to add?

DW: I think finding your own peace of mind is so important. Some people do it with yoga, some people do it with meditative classes. I think even doing a guided meditation from apps work. You can get apps that go through 2-, 5-, 20-, or 60-minute guided meditations.

I find that in 2 to 5 minutes every morning, I can bring myself to a place of gratitude and mindfulness that allows me to create energy instead of stress.

The butterfly meditation got me to this place where I was feeding myself versus letting so much feed off me. I went through this meditation before I went to sleep, and it allowed me this peace of mind to fall asleep and then get up in the morning and do the same thing. When my antenna is going crazy and I'm feeling stressed, I'll just go into a mindful meditation for 2 minutes where I fill myself up with positivity and light, and go out and give it away.

Finding what resonates with you is really important for not only the physical aspect, but the mental aspect of it.

Find your bliss.

Please note: the transcript of this interview has been edited.

Survivor Interview: Pam Hendrickson

Pam Hendrickson is one of my dearest friends. She, her husband, Chris, my wife, Vivian, and I have been through crazy things together. Our kids were born 6 months apart, and we have a business together. Pam and I have co-created many products. For 18 years, she was responsible for creating the majority of Tony Robbins' products. She's an incredibly bright and talented person and a thoroughbred workhorse.

Not long ago, I received "the call" from Chris—there's a lump in Pam's breast. After lots of tests, the results came in ... cancer. As of the writing of this book, Pam has gone through surgery and is undergoing chemotherapy. The photo below was just taken of Pam—with her very cute recently-shaved head.

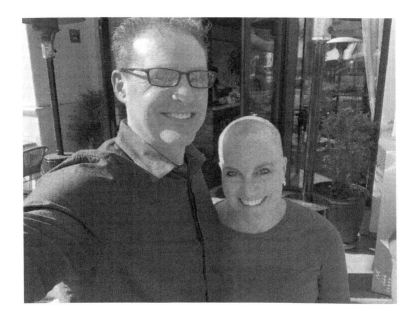

Mike Koenigs: How did you find out you have cancer?

Pam Hendrickson: A routine mammogram. It was the last thing I was expecting. If you would've given me a list of 50 things that could've been wrong with me, this was number 50. I don't have any risk factors. I live a pretty clean life.

It was a routine mammogram, and the tech was awesome. She actually felt the lump and said, "What you got going on here, girl?" That led to about 40,000 tests and then the diagnosis.

MK: From the time it showed up, what were your first thoughts and concerns?

PH: Honestly, I don't think I believed it. Until the doctor came in to read the ultrasound in front of me, I don't think I believed it. Number one, there's so much going on in our bodies. It could be so many things. I think second, it's that whole, "Well, this isn't going to happen to me." I thought it was going to be something benign.

Eight days later I went in for the ultrasound. The ultrasound tech called the MD to look at the ultrasound. But the tech knew. They've seen millions of these. She said, "Look, you need to confirm it, but I've seen a lot of these, and I can tell you it doesn't look good."

I can remember sitting there, the exact bed, the stupid little blue and purple chandelier thing that was above the bed. You just remember every little detail of that moment.

MK: What, in order, were your biggest concerns?

PH: The biggest is shock, like, "What?" Then I was worried about my husband. He hadn't been thinking there was going to be anything. I was thinking, "My gosh, how am I going to tell all my family?"

I know in my life a lot of times when something happens, I immediately go to the worst, and then it ends up not being as bad. This is such a crazy situation because I went, "It's not that bad," and then every single test we did, it got worse. It was kind of a surreal thing that way. Maybe that was good for me to experience something differently like that and still know everything is okay, but I still didn't believe it was that bad.

MK: There are some people that think the causes of cancer are environmental, then there's dietary, and then there's genetic. Louise Hay talks about the emotional causes of cancer. You may have an instinctive feel for what you think may have caused it. Is it environmental, dietary, genetic, or emotional? Or a combination?

PH: My gut reaction 100% is emotional. I think when anything happens, a person's first response is getting upset. Then as you start to think about it, you have to look at how you contributed and what needs to happen differently moving forward.

That's really hard. It's hard to do that honestly. It's easy to do it in a way that either you give the answers you think everybody wants to hear. It's harder to get the real answers, but I think in my case it had an emotional root.

MK: You find out, "My body has cancer. I'm going to be going down a pathway of treatment. This may be a year long." What went through your head in terms of your biggest concerns, fears, and communicating this both to your family and to your clients?

PH: What's interesting is that I didn't know what I didn't know. I don't think I really knew it was going to be the ordeal that it's been.

Some of the advice we got early on was "It's just a little thing. You just have a little mastectomy, and it's fine." Three months later, it's like, "Okay, it's widespread to your entire breast. It's in your lymph." That, I think, affected our feelings about it differently.

Chris is great. He and I have had our issues. We're both very emotional people, as you know, yet when big things happen, I think we tend to come together better. In a weird way, we did. We talked about it. We're like, "We've got to make sure we're great when this is all over."

He was upset. I think I was surprised at how upset he was. He cried. He was very upset. That really disconcerted me more than even my own upset. I expected him to be upset, but I just didn't expect his reaction quite at that level.

I don't think we told the children until the biopsy came back. Until the biopsy comes back positive, even if you are pretty sure, you don't know 100%. We decided we wanted to wait until we knew for sure. It was so funny because you get a lot of people who want to give advice unsolicited. Everybody has an opinion, right? "You can't tell your kids," and others, "Yes! Tell your kids everything."

For us, what made sense was to tell them, but to not give them every excruciating little detail.

For me growing up, I was really protected. My parents didn't share bad things with me. That really, in retrospect, wasn't a good thing. It didn't teach me how to be prepared to deal with that stuff. I just think for our kids, it's just part of life.

Fortunately for our kids, they have the reference of you, Mike. They know that you walked out okay. That was a huge help because they had a reference.

We told them individually because we wanted them both to have the space to respond how they were going to respond, versus playing off each other as siblings do. We just told them very matter-of-factly. We tried to not make promises we couldn't make, like that it's treatable. We said something like "There's every reason to believe that this thing is treatable, and then we can rid of it. There's no guarantees in life, but your mom is a tough lady and we're going to get through this. We're going to need your help."

Along the way, we told them major things, but again, we didn't tell them every little detail. There was a 2.5-week period where my bone scan and PET scan came back positive on my hip. Usually if both of them come back positive, it's not good. Usually that means bone metastases. We didn't know. I needed a bunch more tests. You're always waiting for tests.

During that period, we're like, "Fuck. What if this is bone metastases? It changes everything." We didn't tell them any of that. They didn't know until we were through it because until we knew, there was no point. I'm glad we didn't because it turned out I've got some other benign thing in my hip that's not, thankfully, cancer.

MK: You've been exposed to holistic medicine and integrative therapies. You've got your band of docs. What treatment protocol have you decided to do?

PH: What I've learned is it's just so different for everybody, and it's so personal for everybody. We took time to research, and I'm so glad we did.

Jeremy Geffen's best advice is when you find out you have cancer, step number one is slow the fuck down. That was really our mantra for the first month because it's hard. When you find out you have it, you're just like, "Cut it out! Let's go in tomorrow for surgery. Just get it out of there." That would've been such a mistake because we didn't have all the data. We wouldn't have cut out enough. We wouldn't have cut out the right things. I think that was really our mantra. God bless Jeremy. That's a big piece of his legacy he left for us: slow the fuck down.

We researched. We went up and met with doctors. We met with Dr. Delaney. We met with our psychotherapist. We met with medical doctors. We met with 3 different medical teams.

What was crazy is when you're diagnosed, they just assign you doctors. Most people just take the doctors they are assigned. We met with a surgeon who is great, but breast is only 30% of what he does. In my mind, I'm like, "No, no, no, no, no, no, no, no, no. I need somebody who this is all they do." Kind of like the Terminator. This is what he does. It's all he does. That was just our mindset. We needed somebody who did breast only and was super current in breast.

It took a while and it took a lot of money because you pay for every bloody appointment, whether you use the doctor or not. In the meantime, we're getting tests. You take a test and you wait for 5 days, 7 days, 10 days to get the test results back. Those damn biopsies take forever, but I'm really glad we did it. Looking back, my surgery was delayed 3 weeks later than we wanted it to be, but it didn't change anything, and we had the right doctors.

My treatment, my medical team, at that phase of my treatment, certainly were working with Dr. Delaney to help me. I think where she really helped me was to take a lot of integrated stuff to help me get ready for surgery and be strong for surgery. I feel like in many ways, I was stronger physically and mentally before I went into surgery than I had been in a long time.

Tony Robbins had given me a referral as well. Very similar, all integrative health people. I used that to get strong for surgery.

Right now, I'm in a medical phase. In the medical phase, it is my medical doctors. They have an answer for everything. I'll bring up integrative ideas or concepts, and they have an answer.

I was planning to take all my antioxidants to chemotherapy, and again, this might not be right for everybody, my doctor pointed out, "Why would you do that when the whole point of chemo is to oxidize stuff? If you're taking too much antioxidants, you're counteracting what the chemo is trying to do."

My medical team has been phenomenal, and they're just so up on the research. I haven't found anybody else as up on the research. They've successfully cured this. I kind of don't want to hear from somebody who has ideas or thoughts or "I think this works" or "My Aunt Susie's brother's cousin's nephew's brother went to Mexico and did a treatment, and it was amazing." I want a doctor who does this all day long and has cured not just one person, but thousands of people with my exact same conditions. That's what I feel like we have and that's awesome.

Once I'm done with the chemo and the radiation, and especially the chemo, then it's time to rebuild, pack up my body; then Dr. Delaney's stuff will come more into play.

I'm exercising like a banshee. That is the one thing I'm doing. He says the number one thing I can do to combat feeling lousy during treatment and also for recurrence for breast cancer is exercise. It is known to be one of the top things you can do to prevent recurrence, so I am doing that.

Some chemo drugs you lose your hair. Some you don't, right? There's something called a "cold cap" or a "penguin cap" that you can use to freeze your scalp while you're getting chemo. You can often preserve a lot of your hair that way. My first response was "Of course I would do that. Why wouldn't I preserve my hair?" When you talk to these oncologists, it makes total sense. The way it works is it freezes your scalp, so the chemo isn't getting up into your scalp.

Probably the cancer didn't get into my scalp. However, If you're going through chemo, why would you do anything that would prevent the chemo from getting anywhere in your body as important as your brain? That was my mindset: "Yeah, I don't want to lose my hair, but I don't want cancer in my brain even more."

Like I said, the exercise has been really good for me. It's disgusting. I just smell myself sweating out of it. Neuropathy has been awful. The only thing that combats it is exercise.

MK: Let's talk about your business. What's going on there?

PH: I've worked like a dog for almost 30 years now, and we just made a decision. My husband's mantra is "You have one job right now and that's to get better." We've been paying SDI, state disability, for many years. We are on disability right now.

I have a very small team. They're awesome, and they've been so supportive. They're running my online business. I wouldn't say we're growing my online business, but we're certainly maintaining it and keeping enough money in there to keep it going.

I've got very understanding people and clients, consulting clients, and customers, here and there. It's been a wild thing. I'm really not doing much.

MK: If you're looking at from the moment you got word— and you've been consulting with doctors, with non-doctors, with integrative, with friends, family, etc.—what's the best piece of advice you've received from anyone about cancer so far?

PH: It's a couple things. I think number one is that it's an ultimate opportunity to restructure your life. If you don't take any life crisis as an opportunity to restructure things, then you're missing the point. When I say "restructure," it means emotional and physical relationship changes. It means work and doing what you really love to do.

David Cassidy died recently, and I read an article about how unhappy he was. He never got to live his dream. I just thought how lucky we who have cancer are because it's an opportunity for renewal. It's the greatest gift.

My husband has bought me so many little gifts, and my favorite one is this little baby Groot from *Guardians of the Galaxy*. He said, "This is about new beginnings." I think that's it.

I'm about to go buzz cut my hair. I know I'm going to sob like crazy. In some ways, it's just the ultimate symbol of a new opportunity. I think you have to look at it that way. It's life. It sucks, it's hard. I think you realize you're so much stronger than you thought. Quite honestly, I am amazed at how physically and emotionally strong I am. I always knew I was a strong person, but like everybody with cancer, I've dealt with a lot of physical and emotional stuff.

I think the big advice is listen to those whispers of destiny and restructure.

Another mantra Chris and I have is "We're blessed." We've reconnected at a deeper level with so many family and friends, and that's just been beautiful. I don't really listen to Tony Robbins, but if you're going to take in the bad, you've got to take in the good and you've got to take in the beauty.

I think sometimes cancer is a result of no longer taking in the beauty. We stopped seeing the beauty that's already around us. I think cancer is an opportunity to reawaken yourself to the beauty that is there, that maybe you've been missing.

Please note: the transcript of this interview has been edited.

About Mike Koenigs

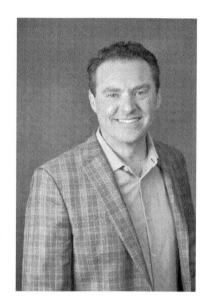

Originally from tiny Eagle Lake, Minnesota (population 763), Mike barely passed high school, never went to college, but taught himself how to program and write video games when he was 14 to escape his small-town roots and become a serial entrepreneur, building software and training programs to help entrepreneurs get attention to get found, seen, heard, watched, and read on any device, anytime, anywhere, and on demand.

For Mike, it's not all about the money—he's raised over $2.4mm for his wife Vivian's Just Like My Child foundation. He's also a stage 3a cancer survivor, completing 9 months of chemotherapy and 33 radiation treatments. His doctors say he's healthy and cancer-free.

He's a 13-time #1 bestselling author, "Marketer of the Year" winner, serial entrepreneur, filmmaker, international speaker, and patented inventor. His products have simplified and automated marketing for over 54,000 small businesses, authors, experts, speakers, coaches, and consultants in 121 countries.

Mike built and sold his last two businesses to publicly traded companies, including his most recent exits, Traffic

Geyser and Instant Customer. His first company, Digital Cafe, was sold to the publicly traded Interpublic Group.

He lives on the beach in La Jolla, San Diego, with his wife and son, Zak.

He can be reached at his personal website at www.MrBz.com or business site at www.YouEverywhereNow.com.

Twitter: @MikeKoenigs

Facebook: www.Facebook.com/Koenigs (Fan Page)

www.Facebook.com/MikeAKoenigs (Personal)

Meet Mike—watch his sizzle reel here: www.YEN.tv/Sizzle

Book Mike Koenigs to Speak

Book Mike Koenigs as Your Keynote Speaker and You're Guaranteed to Make Your Event Inspirational, Motivational, Highly Entertaining, and Unforgettable!

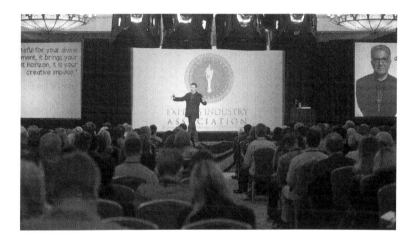

For over two decades, Mike Koenigs has been educating, entertaining, motivating, and inspiring business owners, entrepreneurs, authors, experts, speakers, consultants, and coaches to build and grow their businesses with online video, social media, mobile, and product creation strategies.

His origin story includes his recent near-death brush with stage 3a cancer, growing up lower middle-class in a small town in Eagle Lake, Minnesota, with severe ADHD, and "meeting" Tony Robbins through an infomercial that changed his life forever. After successfully building and exiting from two companies and selling them to publicly traded companies, Mike can share relevant, actionable strategies that anyone can use—even if they're starting from scratch.

His unique style inspires, empowers, and entertains audiences while giving them the tools and strategies they need and want to get seen and heard to build and grow successful sustainable brands and businesses.

For more info and to book Mike for your next event, visit www.MrBz.com/Speaking OR call or text +1 (858) 412–0858.

Will You Leave a Book Review?

Did you enjoy this book and find it useful?
I will be very grateful when you post a short
review and give your success story on Amazon
right now!

Your support makes a difference. I *read and
respond to all the reviews personally* to make this book
even better!

To leave a review right now, go here:
www.YEN.tv/CancerpreneurReview

Endorsements and Accolades

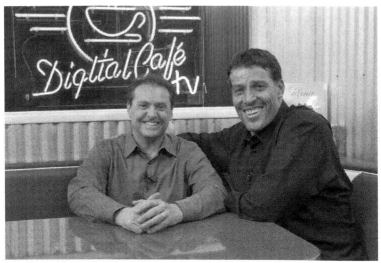

Mike is an extraordinary man. He's brought me insights on how to reach people on the Internet that are incredibly valuable. This is a man you should deal with. Take advantage of what he has to offer.

—Tony Robbins, World Authority on Leadership Psychology and the Nation's #1 Life and Business Strategist

There are those who lead and those who follow, and then there are trend-creators. Mike is a true leader who uses his creative genius and relentless pursuit of new frontiers and technologies to change the landscape of what

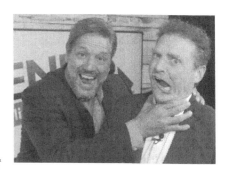

is possible and usable in today's crazy, ever-changing business landscape.

—John Assaraf, NYT Bestselling Author and CEO NeuroGym.com

Mike Koenigs is the "Doc Brown" of marketing automation and technology. One question or problem unlocks his brain and 20 to 30 ingenious ideas pour out of it. One idea grew my database from 30,000 to 800,000 in 14 months. 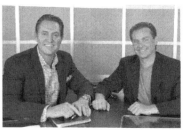 *Another one contributed to a product launch that generated a million dollars in three days. Most recently another contributed to a marketing automation process that is now generating $250,000 a week. So yes, like "Doc Brown," if you can get past the crazy outfits and wild hair, Mike Koenigs is a brilliant marketing muse that can make you money!*

—Darren Hardy, Founding Publisher/Editor SUCCESS Magazine and Mentor to CEOs and High-Performance Achievers

I feel very blessed to have Mike Koenigs as a friend and in my personal and business life. After many years of teaching people around the world, it is guys like Mike Koenigs that keep me 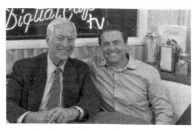 *sharp. And we both share the same goals of wanting to help millions of entrepreneurs achieve their goals to greater financial and business success. More people need to engage in Mike's teachings—quite amazing!*

—Brian Tracy, Author, Speaker, and Entrepreneur

About Cancerpreneur

According to the American Cancer Society, an estimated **1,688,780 new cancer cases** and **600,920 cancer deaths** will occur in the US this year. According to the US Small Business Administration, 9% of the US population are small business owners and entrepreneurs. That means over **150,000 small business owners will be diagnosed with cancer, and more than 50,000 won't survive**, leaving their families, employees, and customers behind.

Until now, there hasn't been a handbook for business owners who are diagnosed with cancer and have to deal with running a business that takes 40–80 hours a week and at the same time caring for a spouse, children, employees, and customers. **This breakthrough book, *Cancerpreneur,* guides the entrepreneur, business owner, spouse, children, employees, and friends through the process of dealing with the complexities of a cancer diagnosis and treatment**.

Stage 3a cancer survivor, serial entrepreneur, and 13-time #1 bestselling author, Mike Koenigs, provides a solution to this complex mess. He successfully survived a cancer diagnosis, treatment, and recovery, while keeping his marriage, relationship with his young son, and business intact. **During his recovery**, he also managed—with the help of his incredible team and advisors—to package and sell his business to a publicly traded company.

As a 5-year survivor, Mike's friends, family, and associates frequently call him for cancer advice. After taking hundreds of calls and giving hours of cancer and health recommendations, suggestions, referrals, and solutions, Mike finally turned his experience and expertise into a bestselling book that can provide entrepreneurs diagnosed with cancer with life-saving strategies.

To learn more and to get free videos and interviews with cancer survivors, visit www.CancerPreneur.com, and find out how to hire Mike as an inspirational keynote speaker or business advisor for your group or organization.

Made in the USA
San Bernardino, CA
16 February 2018